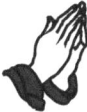 # Soul Wounds
BY DR. KELLIE DIANE
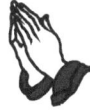

Publisher Awareherness Press Publishers

Awareherness@gmail.com

2nd edition

LCCN 2024919129

ISBN 9781965702017

"What a targeted, detailed approach to healing soul wounds. This book is a page turner that will allow you to see and feel exactly what Dr. Kellie felt as she carefully navigates her journey. The opening questions had me screaming, "This is me!" Dr. Kellie Diane talks about a very transparent journey that led to self-healing, self-discovery, self-vindication, and ultimately self-love. This book will walk you through how to, according to Dr. Diane, "lovingly unpack your baggage," which is needed in order for you to heal in totality. It is not easy to look in a mirror and unpack yourself, but it's much easier to do it to other people. Dr. Kellie shows you just how to do it and heal through it all. After reading this book you should have kicked fear in the face and decided to walk into your future free of bondage and baggage. It's definitely time to heal from the pain of your past." – Chaundra Nicole Gore

"Did I just go back and read this book twice? Yes! AMAZING read. You will not put this book down until you are finished. Kudos to Dr. Kellie Diane for her transparency and dedication to release this book into the atmosphere. Get your soul healed today!" - Susan B.

Are you looking for transparency? This is the book right here. Open it now, read it until the end. Dr. Kellie just blessed my life because I was her. She just helped me in several areas, especially self-esteem. I have already decided to take my life back but now I recommend this book to every woman in need of life changing medication to the soul."
– Ashely Xy

"What? Wait a minute, Dr. Kellie nailed it with this very detailed navigational system all about soul wounds. This book reminds me of Chicken Soup for the Soul has the same caliber of writing. Very well put together and nicely presented." – Brown

"Chapter three made me want to smack those two drivers in the car. Way to go, Dr. Kellie Diane, for standing strong at four years of age. You ought to be proud of yourself to have conquered that. This was the best chapter in my opinion, but overall, an excellent reading choice.
Very, very good, this will help so many." – Bradley J.G.

"Bravo, Dr. Kellie Diane! This book was written for all those women that need deep healing. This book walks through your life and mine, too. Very eye-opening, real-life situations that make you want to stay silent. Bless your heart for taking the time to write your power out in words. I read this book in 1 hour from beginning to the end. Very great book." -Waverly B.L.

"Excellent walk through her life. This book will change lives forever. A must read until the very end. Don't stop until you get to the last word. Dr. Kellie is saving you some time." - Beatrice B.

"Our pain is necessary. Dr. Kellie reminded me of that as I walked through her journey, Soul Wounds is an action-packed movie on paper. Bravo, Dr. Diane, Bravo!" -Seth. W

"Very quick read, that made me cry for the most part. It sparked something in me to take care of me. I would say it can be developed a bit more in a few areas, seems like there is more to the story, it left me hanging. Great storyline." – John G. Jame

Soul Wounds

🙏 Dedication 🙏

To the Author and Finisher of my Life, The ONE and ONLY TRUE GOD. Thank You for constant guidance, love, and protection. Thank You for NEVER leaving my side and for showing me who I was divinely created to be in You. Thank You for gifting me with PURPOSE and DIVINE INSPIRATION. There is NO ME, WITHOUT YOU.

To my children; Jessica, Whitnee, Kevin, Kellee, and Camden. Thank you for choosing me as your mother. For coming into the world to show me what true love really feels like. For trusting me when I was unsure of what the road held ahead of us. For inspiring me when I could not find the strength to inspire myself. My hope is that in healing my wounds you will begin to heal yours. That you will continue to shine even when the world attempts to dim your light. That you will always trust your inner being, your God-self, and never doubt your intuition. I love you.

To my grandchildren; Omari, Elijah, Sterling III, Genesis, Makai, Journey and Jade. My GRAND-GIFTS. It is your time to shine. The world is waiting on your leadership. Embrace who you are and never doubt the amazing path that God has prepared for you. ALWAYS follow the light. I love you always

To my best friends; Marla S. Mckinney and Monaye Rikard. Thank you for being the constant shoulder for me to lean on without judgment. Thank you for walking through this journey with me as my constant cheerleaders. Thank you for never allowing me to give up in my darkest hours. For always reminding me to look to the hills from which cometh my help. Thank you both for always believing in me. I love, love, love you both.

To *my siblings*. We made it through. We had a rough start, but here we are. Evolved and making strides in the world that counted us out. I love you guys. WE GOT THIS!

To my parents; David and Sandra. Thank you for showing me HOW TO LIVE LIFE. Thank you for giving me opportunities that would have been missed had you not embraced me as your own. I thank you for so unselfishly sharing your life with me and helping me develop into the woman that I am today.

To my biological parents, Magnolia and Simmy. Thank you for GIVING ME LIFE. I love you. Rest with God.

To all my countless friends and family who pushed me to be my best, thank you for all your words of encouragement.

And finally, TO MY INNER CHILD! I'm back. I had to protect you, but I'm NEVER leaving you again. You are SAFE NOW! I love US!

Table of Contents

🙏 Acknowledgements 🙏

To all of the beautiful brave souls who have decided to take the journey to heal their wounds and purchase this book, thank you for supporting me on this endeavor.

Thank you to my beautiful granddaughter, Genesis, for lending your beautiful picture to my book cover to make my vision come to life.

Thank you to my handsome grandsons, Sterling and Makai, for being a part of the video visual for this book release.

Thank you to my siblings, Audrey, Kevin, and Corey who constantly support my vision and encourage me to fulfill my dreams. I love you to the moon and back.

And finally, thank you to my little fur babies, Reds, Snowball, Angel, Sage, Willa Mittens and Brownie, who so graciously greeted me at the door, licked my wounds, and walked by my side in this life.

🙏 Foreword 🙏

Throughout our lives, we encounter many people, obstacles, and challenges that force us to reach deep to tap into our most basic survival skills. Every once in a while, we come across someone or something that acts as a beacon of light to assist in our navigation of these challenges (life's peaks and valleys). I consider Dr. Kellie Diane to be one of those beacons of light. For 25 years, I have witnessed first-hand, Dr. Diane rediscovers the light she possesses. After each of her life struggles, she stood even stronger. Always learning and growing along the way. As her light gets brighter, she never ceases to reach out, lift, and empower other women. Women who may have forgotten that their light comes from within, not from any outside relationship or experience (source or soul wound).

Soul Wounds takes the reader on a journey through, enlightenment self-awareness and healing. The lessons taught in this book speak to the brokenness we all suffer from time to time in our lives. Through relatable life experiences, Dr. Diane reveals pearls of wisdom that every reader can use as a guide through this quagmire we call life. She reminds us about the importance of self-love and forgiveness and that we are all redeemable. Dr. Diane reveals how to identify the 5 Soul Wounds that shape, mold, and direct our lives and how to use them to overcome. Let us reclaim our power! In the words of the author, "Grab your tea or coffee and snacks. We've got work to do, baggage to lovingly unpack, and wounds to heal!"

Enjoy!

Marla S. McKinney

Educator, Spiritual Advisor, Seeker of Truth, and Life-Long Friend.

🙏 Introduction 🙏

Healing begins the moment you decide to take your power back by healing your wounds. One of the most important relationships that you will ever have is with yourself. True love is found by going within yourself and then it radiates out into the world. You must be brave enough to heal the pain that threatens to constantly dim your light and dull your shine. You were designed to shine. Congratulations on the journey to the new you!

It is said that hurt people hurt people.
"I'm going to get them before they get me."
"I hurt you because you hurt me."

Have you ever found yourself making these statements? Have you ever found yourself overreacting to situations that appear at first to be seemingly small? Have you ever had a sudden mood swing after having a regular conversation with a friend, family member, significant other, or associate? Have you ever walked away from a seemingly innocent conversation feeling a sense of void or pain? Have you ever overextended yourself only to have the same energy not given back to you? Have you been on a rollercoaster of toxic relationships, one after another? Have you ever felt the need to

16

always be in a relationship because you were afraid to be alone? Have you remained in relationships even though you were being abused and mistreated? Do you have a difficult time trusting people?

Pour your coffee, sip your tea, and grab a snack. We have work to do. We have baggage to unpack lovingly. We have wounds to heal and conquer. It is time to heal so that the future generations that we are gifted to birth or encounter inherit our healthy thought processes. Let us transition from brokenness to wholeness by healing generational traumas. Let us take our power back by having healthy, transparent conversations and loving ourselves unconditionally. When we feel good enough to love ourselves, then others will love us, too.

I remember being in the darkest place of my life. A place that I did not know how I was going to come out of or how it was going to end.

I knew that I was going to come out of it, I just did not know what shape I was going to be in when I did. My faith was in God. I knew that God would deliver me out of it eventually. One day I realized that I kept repeatedly dealing with the same demon that manifested in different faces. They left me feeling hurt and defeated. I had gotten away scathed, but barely alive. I was chipped, not broken, but nevertheless, alive. I had somehow once again ended up in a rabbit hole that I vowed to never go down again in life. That cold, winter day, out of breath and spiritually bleeding, I pulled together every ounce of energy that I could garner within me and ran for my life.

"God, I promise you that if you pull me out of this rabbit hole and heal my heart, I will never go back."

I decided at that point in my life that no matter how much it hurt, I was going to heal my pain and get off the hamster wheel of constant dead ends. I concluded that the common denominator was me and that I was doing something vastly wrong. I had no idea what I was doing wrong; all I knew was that I was willing to overturn every stone to find an explanation to end the constant nightmare of hurt after hurt. On this day, distraught, wounded, and feeling the worst emotional pain imaginable, I decided that I wanted to take my power back. I wanted to live.

My truth is that the entire time I thought I was falling apart, I was falling together. The puzzle pieces to my life were falling into place strategically. One by one. As I picked them up, I realized that the full picture was so much brighter than I could have ever imagined. I was on a journey in which I had forgotten to appreciate that each battle was designed for me to win the war that was within me. The war that constantly screamed that I was not good enough, smart enough, or pretty enough. The war that screamed that I was unloved and unwanted. The war that ended when I decided to love myself unconditionally and walk in my power. The result of the war was that I had discovered myself.

It has often been said that the truth starts with a conversation. The most important conversation that you may ever have is with yourself. The conversation when you decide that what you are doing in your life is no longer effective. It is no longer manifesting the results that are satisfactory to your liking. I am writing this book just to let you know that you can come out of it. You can come out of it healed in a different place then where you were when you went into it. You can come out of it with hope and a renewed spirit. You do not have to remain in this place, it is a place that is temporary. It is not a place that is designed for you to stay for a long time. It's simply a pause in the magnificent path of your life. A pause so that you can take time to reassess and reframe what you want your life to look like. A pause to rewrite the script of your life and tell your truth. This is the time to address the wounds that sat silently in the background causing you to slowly die a slow death of untold truths and misconstrued ideations.

It's time for you to discover YOU.

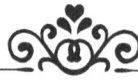

Chapter One
What are Soul Wounds?

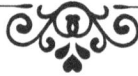

🙏 Many secrets are 🙏
hidden in the basement
of your soul, still weeping.

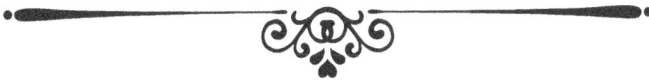

🙏 Healing requires you 🙏
to UNLEARN what was
taught to you as a child and
relearn who you REALLY are.
Your power lies WITHIN!

I am your sister, your aunt, your mother, your coworker. I am the doctor that you see every year, your lawyer that defends you in the courtroom, and your neighbor who wears a bright smile every morning when you greet them. When you look at me, who do you see? What do you see? Do you see fear, depression, or perhaps anger? Perhaps you see a strong, confident woman who is ready to conquer the world. A woman who has all her little duckies in a row, a woman who has led a perfect life. Quite frankly, I could be all these things, some of these things, or none of them at all. I could even be you! Who am I, you ask? I am one of many individuals who has carried an unhealed Soul Wound around for most of my life. Living my life on autopilot, unable to deal with all the Soul Wounds that were inflicted on me early on in my childhood. I was merely dealing and not healing. Wake up, repeat. Then wake up and repeat again. I felt as though I had conquered them because I had survived them. However, one day my life came to an abrupt halt because my baggage was too heavy to travel another step, leaving me to deal with all my wounds. Wounds that had temporarily robbed me of the person that God had designed me to be before I was born. Wounds that ripped me to my core, that left me empty, ashamed, lonely, and partially defeated. Wounds that had remained nameless throughout my life but quite destructive. These wounds that I unintentionally discovered are called Soul Wounds.

A *Soul Wound* does not discriminate. It affects all sexes, ethnicities, and nationalities. It comes with a powerful punch with intentions of stealing your joy and robbing you of your potential. A Soul

Wound is a wound that was inflicted on us as a child that caused so much trauma to our soul that it impacted every area of our lives. The wound was so injurious that even as an adult, it affects everything we do and everywhere we go. It affects your decisions, your moods, and the lens in which you now view your life. You may have even been walking around with wounds your entire life, wondering why you are triggered in certain situations. Why do you feel angry inside towards certain situations? Why do you feel uncomfortable in other situations even though others around you appear to be amazingly comfortable?

These wounds were probably inadvertently produced because of the pain that someone else in your life experienced. The pain that someone else had not taken the time to heal before they gave birth to you.

Sometimes people do not even know that they are causing these traumatic injuries. They are in so much pain in their own lives that they just project whatever is on the inside on the outside. The blame is placed onto you because that person doesn't know how to mend or deal with those wounds. Sadly, some individuals with Soul Wounds feel as though they should not even be addressed and they start to live their lives through the lens of those wounds. They begin to lose trust in themselves gazing through their obscured lens. Regretfully, they continue to move on through life unconsciously refusing to address the deep-seated wounds because they believe that it is never going to get better. These wounds are called abandonment, injustice, betrayal, rejection, and humiliation. The key to healing these wounds is to first acknowledge that you have them, identify what wounds are affecting you, and accept that there will be tons of work to do to heal them.

Understand that this is a journey, not an event; it is an arduous process. This journey is going to take time, truthfulness, and probably lots of tears. However, understand that for you to rescue yourself you must go deep down inside to find yourself and rescue your inner child that has been patiently awaiting you.

Chapter Two
Abandonment

🙏 Only you can rescue 🙏
the child that awaits in
the dark...That child is you!

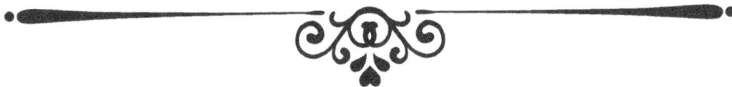

🙏 We were left out, abandoned, 🙏
or perhaps even ghosted. So,
we attach ourselves to anyone
who shows us love even if it is
abusive or toxic. It is better
than being alone, right?

I remember HER. How could I not remember HER? She had a smile that could soften the coldest heart and a voice that could soothe the fiercest storm. She had beautiful, velvety, flawless skin that glowed like a moon's reflection upon a tranquil ocean. I remember wanting to touch her face and lay on her chest. She radiated so much love. She was my mother. My protector. My safe place. My first love. No sooner then I had the chance to know her; she was gone and ripped from my life. I was a little girl roughly around 3, barely out of diapers but an old soul, as some would call it. I was always wise beyond my years but at this moment I was gazing through the eyes of a 3-year-old. I was sitting on the stairs, staring down into the living room between pecan colored balustrade rails. I was observing my mother laugh and embrace a male who was unfamiliar to me. I am unsure if he was unfamiliar because I cannot remember his face or I didn't know who this gentleman was. Was he family, perhaps my father? I was not very interested in who he was, all I knew at the time was that she was sitting on the couch in our house talking to a man who was stealing all the attention away from me She turned around and noticed me glaring and tenderly told me to go up the stairs. Stubbornly, I remained indifferent and continued to watch their interaction. I was a very curious child, I did not talk much. I just watched. It is quite interesting because 50 plus years later I am still the same person; an observer with few words even in the fiercest storm. I was kindly reminded again to go upstairs as I silently peered at the two of them for about 5 more minutes. That was the last time that I remember being in our family home with my mother and the remaining 3 siblings.

I remember the house like it was yesterday. A set of stairs to the left of the entryway which led up to our 3 bedroom and 1 bath modest home. Our home, I now recall, had very minimal furniture but enough for us to remain comfortable as children. I slept in the back room with my brother, who was still young enough to be in a crib. I also had two older siblings who shared a room opposite of mine. I remember that room because that was the same room that a strange man thoughtlessly sat me on the three-story high roof when my mother was out at the store. My guess is that he did not like children and he undoubtedly demonstrated it. My mother found out about it and that was the last time I ever saw him. I recall eating lots of bread for dinner. Feasibly, that is all my oldest sibling could safely prepare because she was barely six years old. My sister was left home alone while my mother was out of the home. She worked effortlessly to feed, protect, and care for her three younger siblings, who at the time were four, two, and under a year of age. A baby herself, my sister kept us alive until our mother came home. Sometimes, mother did not return home at all. The one day that she did come home, she arrived at an empty home. We were gone, taken by the Department of Social Services. Unbeknownst to me, this was the first of many journeys that I was about to embark upon.

I remember arriving at this colossal brick house with a beautiful white wrap around porch with a strange lady who I now know was the social worker. The outside of the house had beautiful, evenly cut landscaped bushes that surrounded the home and a freshly cut lawn. The strange lady held my hand as she gently helped me up the stairs one by one. My little legs were much too short to navigate the stairs alone. In her other arm, she swaddled my younger sibling who was wrapped in a tiny blue blanket close to her chest. I remember being greeted by a woman who seemed to be quite excited to have me at her house. She smiled at me, took me by my hand, and walked me through the home. At that time, I did not know whether she was another relative or not. I had seen so many unfamiliar faces in the past few days and equally as many homes.

When I entered the foyer, I saw a beautiful spiral staircase leading to the top floor. I remember straining my neck to gaze at the enormous, heavy yellow curtains hanging from the windows. The curtains looked as though they would never end. I could not fathom how a window could ever be that tall. It was as if I was in a castle like the one I had once seen in a fairytale on television. I stood in the foyer feeling extremely small in comparison to the immense walls that appeared taller than my imagination. I believed that the walls somehow reached the sky, like the tree in Jack and the Beanstalk. The house had a huge dining room and living room with beautiful enormous pictures on the wall and furniture that matched the paint on the walls. I considered that quite possibly I was in a mansion. There were so many rooms on that first floor. The massive kitchen extended across the entire back end of the house, which connected to the other side via a screened in porch. The porch then ended with a spiral staircase that led upstairs to the second level of the home. The bedrooms upstairs were equally massive, with heavy doors that appeared to stand about 18 feet tall. They had clear, crystal-like knobs that I wanted to take off and hide away in my pocket as keepsakes. When I entered one of the rooms, I remember thinking how spacious it appeared. The room itself was more prominent than our entire upstairs at my mother's house. The curtains and windows duplicated the ones on the first floor. It had a huge bed that I ultimately needed help to get into because my legs were much too small even to attempt to do it alone. I remember the new lady tucking me in that night. For the first time in my life, I was in a room alone and I felt it, too. Alone.

As the months and years passed by, I remember spending time with the other foster kids in the home. I quickly realized that they were not very friendly and were not going to make my experience a nice one. I was next to the youngest child there, and apparently, they did not like that I received extra attention. I was quiet, observant, and still did not talk much. My foster mother spent time tucking me in the bed at night and giving me lots of hugs and kisses. I recall waking up in the mornings to home-cooked meals and warm hugs from this new lady. I remember thinking that she smelled really good every time that she lovingly embraced me.

My days were often filled with happiness because every morning my sisters would stop by and pick me up so we could walk to school together. I realized that many times my sisters were very hungry and so my foster mother fed them breakfast as well. They were instructed to not tell their foster mother about the breakfast.

I had no idea back then why this needed to be a secret. All kids eat when they are hungry, right? As an adult I found out that they were not being fed at the home in which they were residing and that their experiences were not at all pleasant.

My happy days at the foster home were numbered as well. Occasionally, my foster mom would go to the store and leave me with the older children. That is when the torture started. They would abuse me for hours. Locking me in concrete covered rooms in the basement in the dark, smothering me close to unconsciousness, and swinging me upside down from the 30-foot spiral staircase. I was threatened after every abusive episode that if I were to tell our foster mother, the violence would get worse. This went on for about 5 years. In return, I stopped talking.

Chapter Three
Injustice

🙏 Even in an empty 🙏
room, they don't see you.

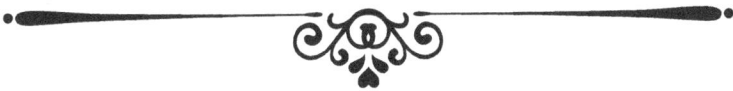

🙏 You were not appreciated or 🙏
valued. Your parents were aloof
or cold hearted. So, you try hard
to be perfect and excel in every
area just so they can see you,
even at the expense of
destroying yourself.

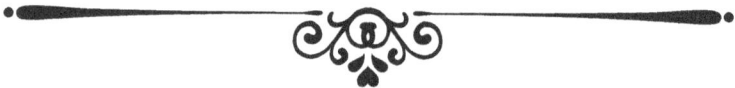

"I think we should just leave them on the side of the road. I bet that would be funny. No one wants them anyway," they said. The two men laughed back and forth as they drove down the road with my brother and I in the back seat. Somehow in my spirit I felt as though they weren't joking, that they were really going to leave us on the side of the road at some point. I remember sitting in the back seat of the car and being incredibly nervous while listening to them. We were traveling down a very dark, winding road with trees on both sides. I was probably around four, not even tall enough to see over the seat, but I could look out the window and see that I was somewhere unfamiliar.

The two guys looked at each other and started laughing and high-fiving each other.

"Yes, we should do that, we should just drop these little orphans off in the middle of the road and see how that feels. I bet they can't find their way home," the driver said. The guy in the passenger seat nodded his head then turned around and looked at me with a smirk on his face.

"I bet you can't find your way back, can you?"

I recall feeling very isolated with no one to shield me. I vaguely recollect the guys being light colored. I thought they were white, but I wasn't too sure. I knew they were related to my foster mother because they had previously been at her home and had spoken to me on numerous occasions. I remember feeling slightly fearful as I watched the two of them converse between each other, talking about executing their plan. Somehow, I knew this was going to happen because I had a premonition about it the night before, so in my mind I already knew what I had to do. A few minutes later, they stopped. They pulled the car over to the side of the road and told us to get out. Being a little child, all I knew how to do was to listen. Doing as I was instructed, I quickly removed my seatbelt.

"Take your little brother with you and get out of the car right now!" the passenger yelled.

As we got out of the car, the male in the passenger seat reached behind him and pulled the door closed. I stood there looking perplexed, holding tightly onto my brother's hand. I was unsure what to do next, but I knew that we had to survive. As I reviewed the plan in my mind that I had established the night before, the car pulled off quickly, leaving gravel, dirt, and dust in the air. I looked as they drove off waiting for them to stop, but they never did. Before long they were way out of sight and we were left abandoned on the side of the road.

I looked around to survey the environment. There were no homes anywhere around and it was approaching dusk. There were trees for miles. Tall, dense trees. I knew that we were miles from home because we had been in the car for at least an hour. I had no idea where we needed to go, but I did know that I needed to keep my brother safe and get him off the road. I held my brother's hand tightly, careful not to let it go as I proceeded to walk in the opposite direction in which we came. I started out walking slowly, holding the small hand of a little one-year-old child who walked as quickly as his little legs could carry him in order to keep up with me. I remember thinking that I needed to keep him on the inner part of the pavement close to the trees so that he wouldn't break away and accidentally run into the road and get hit by a car. My hope was that we would eventually make it back home.

"We could walk for a little while and then find somewhere in the woods to sleep for the night. I can make us a bed from the leaves and lay him on my lap while we sleep and then walk again tomorrow."

I vaguely recalled feeling very afraid because it was dark and the tall trees were beginning to look like tall shadows now. The loud sounds of the mysterious animals no longer felt as though they were my friends and I pulled my brother closer. I imagined it was how Hansel and Gretel must have felt abandoned in the middle of the woods, except we had no food. All of a sudden, my mind flashed to the evil witch in the story and was petrified that she would jump out at any moment, so I hastened my steps. After what seemed like forever, a red car headed in the opposite direction drove up beside us. The occupants in the car were a male and female, and they gave us a very strange look. They looked around and then yelled out the window.

"What are you guys doing out here alone? Where is your mom and dad?"

Though I was extremely shy, I knew that this would probably be our only chance of survival. I shrugged my shoulders.

"I don't know. We are just out here, and I don't know where to go," I replied.

If I remember clearly, the occupants of the car looked quite perplexed to see two little toddlers on the side of the road, one of which was in diapers, trying to attempt to find their way home. The lady looked at the male and then told us to get in the car. Because they were strangers, I was afraid to get in the car. I was not sure what to do. After a few moments, the guys with the black car that we were previously in pulled up, looking quite flushed.

"They're fine," they yelled out of the window. "They are with us. We were trying to teach them a lesson."

They walked over and told us to get in the car. The man and lady looked at them very oddly and shook their heads. The driver of the black car shooed us inside and then proceeded to talk to the occupants of the other car. I did not hear what was said, but the other car drove off, glancing at us over their shoulders. At this point, I was very anxious, my heart was beating fast, and I was on the verge of tears. Everything was a blur; it was dark, and I was cold. I felt as though we were gone forever, and they were never going to find us out in the woods.

As we drove off in the car, the guys started laughing.

"Just where did you think that you were going? You better not ever mention this to anyone, or they are going to take you away, and you will never come back."

The passenger looked at me with a shocked face. I looked at him with tears in my eyes and never spoke a word. All I knew was that I had to protect my brother with everything I had in my little body. I knew that I would do whatever I needed to do for us to survive. It was never mentioned again because, on that day, my soul died. I no longer existed.

One day, my foster mother handed me a piece of paper and told me not to give it to anyone and to keep it safely tucked away. It had my name, address, and phone number on it. I remember her looking sad and having tears in her eyes as I walked out the door with another strange lady. In one hand was my luggage and a small stuffed bear. I remember hugging my sisters and them crying. I had no idea why they were crying. I thought that they were upset because they were not going on the car ride with me. I remember wearing a cute little petticoat that was black and white with a matching bonnet. Though I felt beautiful on the outside; I remember feeling lost, lonely, and afraid of what happened so fast in my life. In my first eight years of life, I had been removed from three homes by social services. I was taken from the only safe places that I had known: the arms of my mother, grandmother, and foster mother. I had lost the comfort of familiarity with my family.

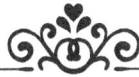 Chapter Four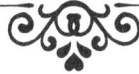
Betrayal

🙏 Hold your head up; your 🙏 crown should never face the ground. Allow it to face the sun so the jewels will sparkle, exposing its brilliance. Like the light that is inside of YOU.

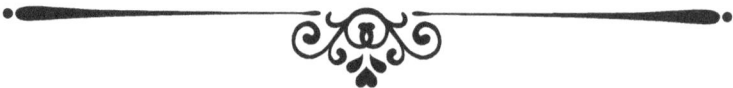

🙏 They told you that they 🙏 would not spank you if you told the truth, but they spanked you anyway. So, as an adult you must control everything. Your mate, your friendships, even your children. If we control everything, no one else can hurt us, right?

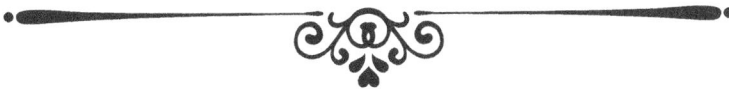

I woke up after what appeared to be an exceedingly long car ride. I do not remember meeting my new family. All that I remember was there was another older male child. He kind of glanced at me, gave me a brief smile and did not say anything else afterward. I, for one, was curious as to whether I was just visiting again or if I was going to remain there for quite a few years. This is what I soon discovered would be my new family. The adjustment was extremely challenging. I no longer had the same pleasant experience that I had in my previous home. I no longer saw my older siblings. Somehow, I knew that I did not belong. I was adopted at the age of 8 into another family. I did not know at the time that I was being adopted. Once again, I thought that I was visiting more family.

When I was adopted into my new family, I was introduced to quite a few new family members. As a young child, I thought that they were all extremely nice, but I always felt a sense of emptiness within me. Around the age of 9 or 10, someone did hear me, at least I thought they heard me, and actually cared about how I felt. There was one male family member I found to be extremely attentive and took a special interest in me. I noticed that he would always smile at me and bring me little gifts. He would take me on car rides to the store and buy me whatever candy I asked for. Since I felt as though I would never fit in or be loved, I enjoyed this special attention. I had no idea that his intentions were not good. As a young child, I did not even know what intentions even meant.

As time went on, his hugs got longer and longer as if he did not want to let me go. Then those hugs grew into touching. Touching in places that belonged only to me. One cool fall day, we went for a ride to the store, but he took a detour and took another route. He smirked and told me that he wanted to show me something. I trusted that he had something special for me and waited in anticipation. He told me that the surprise was in the back seat. I got in the back seat hoping that he had a new toy or perhaps some candy hidden beneath the seat. It was in this moment that I learned what true wickedness meant. The man that I trusted had violated me in the worst possible way. I was warned to never mention it.

"Besides, they won't believe you anyway because you are adopted. You don't want to make trouble, or they will send you back," he stated.

I do not remember if we made it to the store that day, but I remember that on that day, another part of my soul died. I could not sort out what happened. He said that he loved me, so it must be right, I thought. It certainly did not feel right. I remember trying to figure out how to make the whole nightmare disappear. A part of me did not want to go back to the foster home and leave my new family, so I decided to keep quiet. However, my nightmare did not end there; it continued. Almost every night, when everyone went to bed, and the lights went out, he crept into my room. He would always firmly remind me of how quickly they could send me back if I ever chose to mention it to anyone. The attacks left me hurt, confused, and ashamed. They continued until I was 13 years old.

The years following were dark, lonely, and rocky. They were filled with suicide attempts, low self- esteem, and brokenness. I did not know who I was or why I existed in this life. It took many years before I saw the light and finally released my pain.

As time passed and I blew my candles out year after year, I slowly realized that my prayers and wishes were going unanswered. No one heard me. No one saw what was happening to me right in front of their eyes. I had no clue what would lie ahead for me in life. They betrayed me; they did not save me. I determined that it was too much churching and no discernment. You know, when you attend church three to four times a week and the saints are so busy pretending to be perfect they cant even discern that one of their own members is hurting.

One day, I decided that I was going to end it all. I no longer wanted to live. I absolutely detested my life. I saw no positive in being on this earth. I remember numbing my wrist in attempts to cut it and take my life. However, after it was numb, God caused me to fall in a deep sleep. It was quite bizarre because I was not sleepy. While I was asleep, a voice which I assume was the voice of God spoke.

"Go back, your work is not done there."

I woke up hours later and it was dark outside. Frustrated that I had fallen asleep, I decided not to take my life that day.

By the time I turned 13 years old, I stopped visualizing a better life.

I stopped making wishes, and stopped fantasizing about a life that was safe and void of hatred and strife. After all, my desperate prayers had fallen on the desolate ground. I started concentrating more on what I was missing from what I believed in for so long. That was my true reality. I started disappearing bit by bit, piece by piece. I no longer saw myself as the little girl with astonishing powers who could change the world. I no longer considered the smiles, hugs, or dreams because they were not manifesting. By the time I was 13, I had been molested, impregnated, and attempted suicide three times. My power had been stolen and my heart had been ripped from my soul. I felt as though I no longer had a voice. My voice was stolen and cast into the sea of the little lost kids. I could not change the world. I could not even save myself.

One day, when I couldn't take the abuse anymore, I decided to tell a teacher who I trusted. I thought about it for some time and decided that day would be the day. I wrote a long, detailed letter to her and asked my friend to give it to her. I remember her coming to the cafeteria and summoning me towards her. I was petrified. I walked slowly with my head down. I no longer had the courage to walk with my head up or the ability to look anyone in the eye. I had been robbed of my essence and my soul was weeping.

"Is this true?" she asked.

"Yes," I nervously answered while gazing at the floor.

"Okay," she responded with tears in her eyes. "I'll speak with someone.

I vividly remember the sympathetic look the teacher gave me when we talked. She talked and I shuddered. I had no voice. I was ashamed, but I had to tell someone. I had to tell someone because I had prayed for months that I wasn't pregnant but knew that I was because I was sick every morning and had cravings every evening. As a matter of fact, he had taken me to a clinic to have a pregnancy test. We left once he found out that the test cost money and that I needed to fill out paperwork. My guess was that he did not want them to realize how young I was and that he was violating me. I remember the individuals in the clinic looking at us real strangely when we walked in there. I now know that they had questions about the age difference. They may have even thought that he was my father. After all, he was 28 and I was 13. I knew that they were going to save me, they had to notice that something was wrong. He quickly took me out of there so that no paperwork was started. They did not save me, either. I felt betrayed.

My teacher told me to go back and try to eat my lunch. My stomach was so upset that I dared not to eat. Following the guidelines of her job, I assumed she subsequently reported it to the principal. It was the first time ever that I felt a small sense of relief. However, I was absolutely horrified. That is the day that my parents found out. It is hard for me, even now, to determine what was worse; the fear of my parents finding out and sending me back or the abuse itself.

I vividly recall the walk to the principal's office. She read the letter that I had written and asked me if it was true. I nodded my head.

She said that she would have to tell my parents and gently sent me back to class. I remember crying silent tears of fear as I watched the clock tick signaling the end of the school day. The ride home on the school bus was the longest drive in my life. This man that was supposed to be my family member had betrayed me and I felt ashamed.

I was brought up in a fairly strict, religious home, attending church quite a few times a week. It was also the era of, "children should be seen and not heard." Our jobs as children were to make our parents proud and do not embarrass them. I believe in my heart of hearts that my parents loved me and did their best to raise and safeguard me from the world. After all, they adopted me by choice and not by force.

As an adult, I feel as though they managed the situation the best way that they knew how. However, what I can say is that it pushed me further into a deep abyss. I was instructed to never speak of the incident again. I never saw a therapist and my feelings were never brought up about the situation. I walked around daily, wanting to disappear. I learned to be noticeably quiet and walk in silence. My body was never mine, and neither were my thoughts. I quietly repeated this over and over in my head. I now know as an adult that when you grow up learning to repress your feelings you do not know how to use them as an adult. When no one listens, you go unheard. You learn not to talk. You learn to suffer in silence and make friends with your pain.

Chapter Five
Rejection

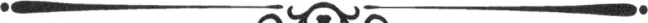
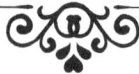

🙏 They can't see the light 🙏
in you because they cannot
see the light in themselves.
Keep shining anyway.

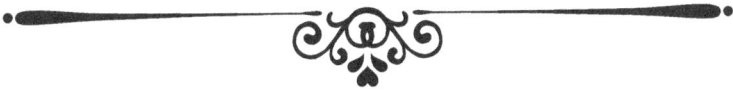

🙏 They prayed for a boy. 🙏 Instead, you turned out to be a girl. So, you grew up, dressed in dark colored clothing so they would not notice you, and constantly criticized your body. You don't matter anyway, right?

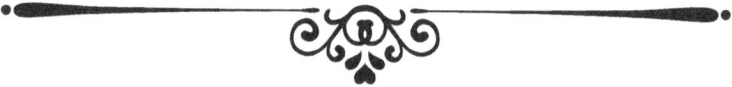

Despite the negative experiences that I encountered as a child, there were some bittersweet experiences, as well. As a family, we traveled often around the country pulling a camper. We belonged to a camping club. We traveled many highways in the back of a jeep with our family dog in tow. I remember each of us fighting over who was going to get the window seat; no one wanted to get stuck in the middle. One day around the age of nine, I won the battle of the infamous window seat and I was enjoying my view. Suddenly, I saw a sign that said,

"Virginia."

I knew that I was born in Richmond, Virginia because I had memorized the address that my foster mother had given me. Perhaps they are taking me back home. I glanced at my parents to observe for any type of reaction. I saw none so I glanced back out the window. My heart skipped in anticipation as we crossed over into Virginia. Roughly around an hour later, I saw a sign that said, "Chamberlyne Ave." Omg, I thought. I am going back to my home. As soon as the sign appeared, it was gone just as fast because they drove right past it.

"Don't get upset, Kellie," I thought. "Perhaps they were going to go another route that I didn't know."

We drove for another 20 minutes, and there was another sign. I saw the big brick building with a clock on the side of the highway that I always remembered as a child. I am surely going home now. My family is somewhere near here, and I know it. But where? As we drove a little further, I began to smell a familiar scent. And then I saw it. It was the Marlboro cigarette building. I screamed inside.

"Yes, I remember this!"

It was the cigarette factory that my elementary school had taken our kindergarten class to tour when I lived with my foster parents. I fixed my clothing and smoothed down my hair in anticipation of seeing my family again. I wanted them to see how I had grown, and I wanted to make a great impression. After all, it had been years. I know that SHE is close by; so is the lady that tucked me in at night! The two girls that walked me to school, too. My father kept driving, head facing the front. No one spoke a word. Slowly, the smell of the Marlboro factory dissipated as we traveled further and further away from the building.

"Why aren't we stopping?" I thought. "My family will be so happy to see me. You are going the wrong way."

The car never stopped, it kept going. The joy was fleeting and happiness continued to evade me. For years, we traveled back and forth on the same familiar highway, which I now know is 95 North, and every time we traveled it, I felt as if needles were being stuck in my back one by one. I lost hope. I silently vowed to return and find my family.

"I will find you one day, I promise. I know that you are out here, but where?"

How could I be so close yet so far?

I remember when my search for my biological family began. I decided one day at work that I would begin the search. I had gotten a job when I was around 17 while in high school. The job required that I called people all over the world to verify crucial information. At that time in my life, cell phones were just a dream and long-distance was billed per minute on your landline. Because it was so expensive, people rarely dialed long distance at home unless it was a dire emergency. I decided that because I had access to a long distance service at work, I would start my search to find my family. I vaguely remembered their faces and a faint remembrance of their names, but I knew that they existed in some form. I had not forgotten who they were. I was much too young to comprehend the relationship status of the two females that I remembered walking me to school in the morning. I recalled that one was of lighter skin than me with an exceptionally long ponytail. She was much taller than me, so I concluded that she was the oldest. I remembered the other one as well, but very faintly. I later was reminded that they lived two doors away from me in another foster home. My mind briefly traveled back to the happy days that I was allowed to eat with them and walk to school as I cautiously dialed the number 8 0 4 ...

I dialed the numbers that I had hidden in my head for the last 10 years of my life.

"Hello?" a feeble voice answered.

"Hi, this is Kellie. You may not remember me, but is this Mama Lydia?"

"Yes."

"It's me, Kellie. Your foster daughter."

"Kellie, is this really you? I can't believe it!"

"Yes, it's me," I replied.

My heart skipped a beat, and I felt tears fall from my eyes. I felt relieved that I was finally beginning to connect the dots. She was real. She really did exist, and it wasn't my imagination.

After staying on the phone laughing, crying, and reminiscing for hours, we began to speak about my siblings and my mother. She told me how she attempted to adopt me, and the state prohibited the adoption because she had become a widow when she had us as children. The state did not think that it would be a great idea to keep us in a single-parent home. By the time that we hung up, I had acquired the name of my older sister. The funny thing was that Mama Lydia was currently babysitting my oldest nephew, which meant that she had remained in contact with my oldest sister ever since I left Virginia. Mama Lydia promised me that she would allow me to talk with my sister that next day when she arrived to drop off my nephew. Since I was under 18, she wasn't allowed to put me directly in touch with my sister. Apparently, if the adoption was closed, it was their rule that my family or foster parents could not contact me until I was 18. I was 17 years old at the time that I contacted Ms. Lydia, but she was able to talk with me since I reached out first.

When I spoke with my sister the next day, she was so happy to hear from me. I, once again, was nervous because I was not sure if she was going to accept me or not. I was not even sure if she remembered me because it had been close to a decade. The conversation ended up being a great one, and she was able to answer many of my questions confirming many of my memories. She also confirmed that I had another sister and a younger brother. My sister was able to give me the name of my father and his last work location that she remembered, but had no further information about his whereabouts. I remember her giving me the name of my mother and verifying that she was alive. For the first time, my heart was whole. I belonged to someone! There is someone out there that loved me and could finally relate to me. I remember thinking, "I wonder if I look like her?" For my entire life, I had been unable to look at anyone who I could say looked like me. I did not care why she gave me up. I just wanted to hug her!

When I finally contacted my mother, she was extremely happy to hear from me. My heart was so filled with joy because I was finally able to hear her voice as I remembered it. That soft, melodic, soothing voice that I recalled when I last saw her at barely three years of age. She was so elated that her baby girl was on the other end of the phone and that I was seemingly okay. She told me how much she loved me and more details about my father. We spoke as long as we could and exchanged addresses and other vital information. Unfortunately, due to the rules that were in place during this stage of her life and some bad decision making, she was currently incarcerated.

Every morning, I was so excited to go to work because I knew that I had an opportunity to continue my search. My next goal was to contact my father. I was able to track him down at a furniture store that he worked at for many decades. I remember calling the store and asking for Mr. Scott and I was put on hold. My heart was beating so fast. What would he say? What would he do? Would he accept me or deny me? My father answered the phone after what seemed to be hours and I identified myself.

"Hello, this is Kellie, your daughter."

After a brief silence he said, "No kidding? I cannot believe that this is you. I always hoped that you would come back and find me." For the second time in my life, I was speechless and felt overwhelming love from a father figure. I thought, "Perhaps dreams do come true."

As we conversed, it was revealed to me that he was married and had been married when I was conceived. He told me the story about how he was unsure if I was his and that he didn't want to take me in when the state asked him to due to his uncertainty. I am guessing that DNA testing wasn't a big thing back then. He apologized for making the decision that he had at the time. He exclaimed that when I was adopted he never expected me ever to show up again. After a few days of phone calls and getting more familiar with each other, he informed me that he spoke with his wife on the day that I initially called and made her aware of the conversation. He invited me to meet her and my paternal siblings. I made him aware that I was not coming into his life to disrupt anything— especially since he was still married. He assured me that it was fine, she approved of the visit, and that I should meet my three siblings. He also informed me that two of my siblings had no idea that I even existed. He and his wife had chosen to keep me a secret.

After talking with my biological family, I decided to meet with them a few months later. I remember feeling extremely nervous but excited to meet my paternal sister. I had never met that side of the family and did not know that they existed. When I met my sister, she looked me up and down as if I were her enemy, like a competitor on the other team. I must admit that I was crushed because I was really looking forward to this sisterly love. Instead, I received a partial embrace. I later discovered that she did not like the idea that I existed because she was a daddy's girl, and up to this point, she believed that she was the only girl. I later met my two brothers, one fully embraced me, but the other refused to even look at me. We went to his job to meet him and I remember him giving me a look of disgust and refusing even to acknowledge me. I then decided that I would never come around again. After all, I had not come to interrupt anyone's family. Throughout my years of yearning and feeling lost, daydreaming about being embraced by my real family, my fantasy of a loving, kind, accepting family quickly came crashing down. I had been rejected by my own flesh and blood.

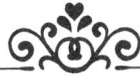

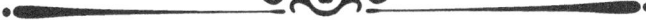

Chapter Six
Humiliation

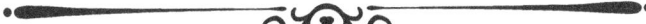

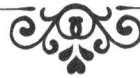

🙏 The right person will 🙏 love you despite your flaws. The wrong person will only love you when you are flawless.

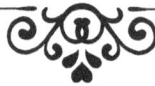

🙏 You couldn't do anything 🙏 right. How dare you embarrass them in front of their friends by spilling ice cream on your clothes at two years old! So, you grow up constantly telling yourself that you are stupid. You are afraid to be seen as selfish, so you overly give in relationships. After all, you should ALWAYS put others first, right?

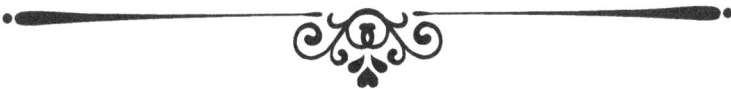

I was living the dream life that I had envisioned for quite a few years. I worked really hard to get to this place in my life. I had a new car, a newly built home, a brand-new husband, and two jobs. I worked a second job out of desire because I loved to have additional money. It was not a necessity, but it was fun to do anyway. I was active in the church and running a marriage ministry. Because I was a registered nurse, part of the job requirement was that I would be on call once every six weekends. This was never a problem for me because I absolutely loved being a nurse and loved my job.

One weekend that I was scheduled to work, I left early with a plan to see all my patients and then return home. The goal was to do my additional paperwork so that I could spend time with my children. I remember leaving one client's home and was on my way to see the last two clients. I was sitting at a stoplight at the bottom of a hill watching the light turn green when BOOM! Suddenly, I woke up and the coffee that was in the coffee holder was splattered all over the car and all over me. I looked up and was startled when a man started knocking on my window. He asked me if I was okay.

"What happened?" I asked

"I didn't see you," he said. I couldn't understand how he couldn't see me or the other four cars that were in front of me but nevertheless I was in too much pain to even begin to process his answer. The cars in front of me were gone and the cars behind me were going around us. I had been rear ended by another vehicle going pretty fast down the hill. This is the car accident that forever changed my life and threw me into my awakening process.

The ambulance arrived at the site to assess me. I remember being in pain all over, feeling as though my body was thrown against a brick wall. The medic suggested that I go to the hospital because my vitals were horrible, but I decided against it. I decided to drive home because the children were still home alone and I did not want them to worry about where I was. When my husband came home from his job, I told him what happened and he took me to urgent care to get further evaluated. The next day I realized that I was in too much pain to work and I was sent home from my job directly to urgent care. When I arrived at urgent care I realized that my condition was beginning to decline. I was given crutches because at this point, I could barely walk on my own.

Throughout the process of multiple medical assessments, it was decided that I was unable to work due to my multiple spinal injuries, so I was forced to abandon both of my jobs. Of course, with me being out of work, that meant that I could spend more time at home doing things to make my marriage a beautiful union. It was an epic failure.

I noticed little things in our marriage that I had not paid close attention to in the past. Yes, there were red flags but due to my abandonment issues, I had chosen to ignore them with hopes that I could fix him. I believed that if I loved him enough and was that

"Proverbs" wife, that he would change. My "Mr. Wonderful" began to change right in the front of my eyes.

I met my "Mr. Wonderful" in February and had gotten married the same year. In hindsight, I realize that it was much too fast to establish a firm foundation with anyone, especially a marriage. He was also am divorcee and had a child with his previous wife. I was overly excited with the thought of becoming a stepmother to another child. He courted me and swept me off my feet. He would come to my house and cook me dinner after I got home from work and take me out on expensive dates. As most couples do, we talked about our past relationships and the possibility of a life together. One day after dating for about 4 months we decided to plan a date out of town. He decided that we should stop by and visit his family since they were in close proximity to where we were headed. After spending about an hour conversing, one of them exclaimed, "Wow, I've never seen you this happy before. When are the two of you getting married?"

Mr. Wonderful quickly responded. "Man, I'm never getting married again."

That should have been strike one, but I disregarded it.

"Me either," I quickly responded.

I must admit that I was a bit disappointed because I was in love and was interested in settling down and getting married. He was a military veteran, had a pretty decent occupation and, was single. I felt as though he was as good as it would get at this point in my life. I had given birth to 5 children from previous marriages and felt as though if he could accept all of us, then what more could I ask for? I was certain that no one would want me at this point. I was determined to show myself and the world that someone wanted me.

As the months passed by, I began to have more in depth conversations with my "Mr. Wonderful." I shared with him my future dreams; how I wanted to become a multi-millionaire and build a legacy. I was at the tail end of achieving another degree and was preparing for the next level in my life of home ownership. I had spent a lot of time speculating how my life would play out if I had a home and I met a guy who also owned a home.

"If I buy a house before I meet a man, I'm not selling my house." I said this in my head repeatedly. I enjoyed my independence and was not willing to compromise it. As luck would have it, my "Mr. Wonderful" happened to be living in his deceased ex-mother-in-law's house and didn't own a home. He apparently had made some type of arrangement with his ex-wife and was paying her rent to stay in the home that was left to her and her sister in the will. This should have been a glaring red flag, but nope. I was too afraid to ask too many questions because I didn't really want to hear the truth and rock the water.

The truth of the matter is once we know the truth, we are obligated to either accept it or make a change. Many of us, in our broken state, chose to not ask questions so that we can remain in our blissful state of what we perceive as love. We literally embrace the statement,

"Ignorance is bliss!"

One day when I was invited to his house, I noticed that he had lots of bottles of alcohol on the shelves in his kitchen.

"Do you drink?" I asked.

"Not really, they belong to my ex. They were left there when I moved in," he replied.

"Oh. Okay." I replied, shrugging my shoulders.

Up to this point I had never seen him drink, so I passed it off as a reasonable response. He was aware that I was not a drinker and had no tolerance for an alcoholic man. Ladies, you have probably gotten tired of counting the red flags so far in this story, but let's be honest, you have done this, too!

On one of our many phone conversations, Mr. Wonderful disclosed to me how his family was having an upcoming family reunion. He expressed his desire to go but couldn't afford to attend the event. He was broke because he was paying child support and couldn't afford any additional expenses. Me, being Ms. Fix It, decided to surprise him with a fully paid trip to the reunion which included the car rental, hotel fees, and gas. He was pleasantly surprised and appeared elated. Why wouldn't he be, he had a fully paid vacation, right?

We loaded the car up on a Friday including 2 of my children, his daughter, and my dog. My other 3 children were already adults and were left behind with their other families. We made the long commute down south and arrived just in time to clean up for the event. When we arrived, we realized that it was an indoor event despite being in a park. Because the dog was with me, I decided to stay outside so that he was not left in a hot car. I tied the dog around the tree and sat down beside him outside as "Mr. Wonderful" and my children walked inside to greet the family. After about 30 minutes a family member realized that I was outside with the dog so they volunteered to watch the dog so that I could eat. Because I didn't want to be a bother to anyone and take them away from their family, I took the opportunity to go in the building to cool off and not eat. I now realize that my deep embedded Soul Wound of abandonment was operating in full effect. I had chosen to deny myself so that I wouldn't be a burden to someone else. Those old feeling of unworthiness crept back in and I took a sit back under the tree, hungry for the remainder of the event. Later that evening after the event came an end, we piled up in the van with plans of going back to the hotel which was about 90 minutes away.

"Are you hungry?" he asked.

"Not right now," I replied. "Maybe I will get something later."

About 60 minutes into the drive, we were close to the hotel and my stomach decided that it wasn't going to wait another minute. "I'm hungry, can we find something to eat?" I asked.

He look at me disgusted. "I thought that you said that you weren't hungry!"

"I wasn't, but I am now. It's no use for me to go to bed starving." I replied.

Immediately the energy in the car changed. I looked over at him and it appeared as if any empathy that he may have had was thrown out of the window. His entire face changed and he looked like he was ready to destroy someone.

"What's wrong?" I asked.

"Nothing. I was going to drop you off and get something to eat," he spat beneath his teeth.

"Well, since you are hungry. Why can't we grab something together while we are out?"

"Because you said that you weren't hungry."

I glanced in the back seat and realized that the children were sleeping. I thought carefully and decided to discontinue the discussion because I refuse to ever argue in front of my children. It was a rule that I had in place before the birth of my first child and had stuck to that rule without any compromise. The rejection wound in me had won. I sat back in my seat and remained quiet as he drove the last 15 minutes back to the hotel.

When we arrived back at the hotel, we unpacked the children and the dog and started to walk inside. I turned around and notice that "Mr. Wonderful" wasn't behind me. He had gotten back into the car and was proceeding to drive off at a high rate of speed. I quickly picked up my phone and dialed his number.

"Hello?"

"Where you going?" I asked.

"I'm going to get something to eat!" he yelled.

"But I told you I was hungry. What about me?"

"I'm going to find something to eat."

"Hello?" I exclaimed into the phone. I heard silence on the other end. He had hung up the phone. I couldn't believe that this man had driven off with no regards to how I felt. I walked upstairs in the hotel, washed up, and tucked the kids in for the night. I waited patiently for my phone to ring, for him to call to see what I wanted to eat.

"There is no way in this world this man is going to get something to eat and not call and ask me what I want."

As the hours passed by, I started to get very upset. I awakened to him climbing in the bed. He appeared much calmer than he was prior to leaving me. I turned my back to him and went to sleep. The next morning there was absolute silence as he moved around me with an uneasy look on his face. We packed the children and the dog in the car after breakfast and proceeded to head home. The entire six hour ride was absolute silence. I was so upset with him that I had decided to leave and never return to the relationship. As we pulled up to my house, he grabbed me.

"I know I've messed up," he said. I looked at him and walked away. Yet again, another red flag.

After about a week we made up and were riding in his car around 11:00 o'clock at night. I notice that his phone started to receive lots of messages. I could tell that they were Facebook messages because of the sound. I looked at him and noticed that he was not checking his phone or even acknowledging that he heard the constant pinging of his phone. I glanced at his phone which was in the cup holder beside me and saw a female's face on the phone.

"Who is this lady and why is she contacting you late at night? Does she know that you are in a relationship?"

"I knew her before I met you." "he replied."

"That's fine, but does she know that you are in a relationship?" He continued to face forward, avoiding eye contact as he drove. "It's obvious to me that she doesn't know that are in a your relationship because she would not be calling you this late at night. I expect you to fix this as soon as possible and don't expect to have this problem again!" I exclaimed. He growled something under his breath and never mentioned it again. Yet again another red flag.

Somehow, after quite a few arguments and multiple red flags, we got engaged. I was hesitant about the marriage but thought that perhaps the marriage would change him into a better man. We decided to get married about a month later at the courthouse. I was extremely nervous.

"Are you nervous?" I asked him.

"No."

We drove to the courthouse where we met my daughter and best friend. My best friend pulled me to the side.

"Do you love him? Because if you don't, we can walk out of here right now and leave."

At this point, I had already exclaimed my love for him to the world and was too embarrassed to back off and walk away. What would people think? Would they laugh at me? If I walk away, it will further prove to the world that I'm a nobody and can't keep a man.

"Yes, I love him," I said. I walked away, returned beside my fiancé, and prepared for the ceremony.

"Repeat after me. I take Kellie to be my lawfully wedded wife, to have to hold, in sickness and health, to death do us part..." the judge stated.

"I take Kellie to be my lawfully wedded wife, to have, to hold, in sickness and health, to death do us part," he repeated with a smirk on his face. The justice of the peace turned to me.

"Kellie, repeat after me. I take this man to be my lawfully married husband to have and to hold in sickness and in health until death do us part."

"I take this man to have and to hold. Hold…" For some reason the words just would not come out my mouth. I attempted to say them two times and stuttered the third time finally getting the words out. When it was all over I had beads of sweat on my forehead. I knew that the moment we were pronounced man and wife that I had made one of the worse mistakes of my life. I had ignored the voice of my inner child and went through with the process. I had betrayed one of the greatest gifts that God had given me. My intuition!

The night of our marriage, we planned to take the kids out to celebrate our nuptials. It was also the weekend of his visitation with his daughter and was super excited to announce to her that we had gotten married. Then the phone rang. It was his ex-wife stating that she would not be able to bring his daughter over until the next day. My new husband was furious. He slammed the phone down and smoke started fuming from his ears. He sat on the bed for hours and didn't move. Not only did we not go to dinner but we didn't consummate our marriage that night either.

"Why are you taking your anger out on me because of what she did?" I asked.

"I'm just mad," he said. Oddly, he remained mad for the next two weeks and refused to touch me. Red Flags!

As time moved on, the abuse became worse. He stopped talking to me all together and would walk past me as if I didn't exist. If that wasn't enough, sex was nonexistent. He would go to bed late and wake up early in order to avoid the act all together. He was constantly whispering something under his breath about his ex-wife and staring off into space with a blank look on his face. He had stated previously that she cheated on him with someone she met online, then subsequently filed for divorce. I couldn't understand why he would be so obsessed over someone who cheated and then left.

The harder he ignored me, the harder I tried to pull him close. The closer I tried to pull him, the worse he treated me. Eventually, I gave him an ultimatum. Either get help or I was leaving. I could no longer live my life the way that it was unfolding in the marriage. I was extremely unhappy. He agreed to seek counseling and I agreed to stay in the marriage. After three marriage counselors and a revelation about a hidden alcohol addiction, the divorce was filed. The man of my dreams ended up being the man of my nightmares. His mask slipped and the real person was standing front and center. I endured emotional, financial, and physical abuse and, of course, there were other women in the picture. I was absolutely devastated.

Throughout the divorce process, the obstacles and misfortunes continued to happen. I had gotten to the point where the headaches that I experienced were so bad that I literally could not lift up my head. The neurosurgeon did additional testing only to find out that the discs in my neck and lower back was destroyed from the car accident. If that was not bad enough, my left shoulder was frozen and I lost usage of my left arm, which was currently in a sling. After careful consideration, the doctor suggested doing both surgeries at one time. The surgery was supposed to be an overnight stay, so I prepared my children for my absence for the next 24 hours. I made sure that they had food and a daily schedule. I was marginally comfortable with them being home without me despite having an alarm system and cameras throughout the home. I had taken the initiative to pay a locksmith a few hundred dollars to change the locks in the home to alleviate my fears from deepening due to my abuse. I was terrified because I had no idea if my ex would return and try to harm my kids. He had been removed due to a temporary restraining order granted by the judge.

I vaguely remember waking up from the surgery with my neck in a brace and my arm wrapped in gauze. I was in a lot of pain and the nurse gave me medication to ease it. After I was stable enough to go to my room for the night, I started experiencing problems. I would fall asleep and stop breathing which would awaken me immediately. I was sent for further testing only to find out that the surgery was causing my throat to close. I was immediately treated for that problem, but the next day I had acquired an infection of unknown origin. The doctor then had to treat me for the infection. Around day 4 of the stay I began to get nauseated and was unable to have a bowel movement. I was sent for testing only for them to find a bowel obstruction.

To make a long story even longer, that one day stay turned into ten days. My only comfort with being away from my children was that I could call them on Facetime or my best friend, Marla, would bring them to visit me. I faithfully checked in on them on the video camera and set my alarm daily to turn the house alarm on and off once they went to bed. Thankfully, I had family members that checked on the children. My uncle also came to the house with enough food to feed a crowd to make sure the kids had plenty to eat. Eventually, I finally made it home with what was the beginning of multiple surgeries. This was the first of seven surgeries in less than four years.

After the first two surgeries, it was time to go to court to finalize the divorce. It ended up being a very nasty divorce filled with lies, scandals, and the loss of my new home. My name was scandalized, my e-mail and bank accounts were broken into, and a relationship with a family member was sabotaged. I had enough and was desperate to get out of the marriage. I told the judge that I would do whatever it took to get out of that marriage. All I wanted was my name back. I walked out of the courthouse a newly divorcee. Within a few hours I found myself in critical condition in the hospital.

I decided that I wanted to celebrate my divorce by not cooking. I walked into the pizza shop and immediately felt extremely cold and dizzy to the point of not being able to stand. I decided that I would attempt to drive home, which was less than a mile away. I gave the children pizza and I climbed in the bed. I felt like death as pain filled my body. I did everything I could to get warm but nothing worked. I was under two huge blankets and a sleeping blanket, and I just could not get warm.

The next morning, the ambulance was at my house, and as stubborn as I am, I knew not to resist the care. Once I arrived at the hospital, the doctors ran multiple tests to find out what was wrong. The last test came back and the doctors entered the room looking extremely nervous.

"It's a growth in your abdomen," they said. "A mass, and it could be cancer."

At this point I was too sick to even care to live. Absolutely exhausted from the struggle of the divorce, I was ready to go home to be with "God". After being transferred to a bigger hospital and given three units of blood immediately, the doctor stated that I had to have emergency surgery. She stated that had I not come in that I would have probably not made it another day. After careful consideration I decided to go home after being stabilized a few days so that I could get the kids prepared for me to have emergency surgery. I did the pre-op testing for surgery and found out the mass was non-cancerous but needed to come out nonetheless or I would end up in critical condition again. For the third time in two years, I had almost died. I was dependent on people to do everything for me. I had lost my dignity, my love for myself, and my willingness to know where to begin again. I felt as though the world had watched me soar and fall down just as suddenly.

I was absolutely humiliated. I had given every part of me to the point of having nothing left for myself. I tried to be everything for everyone and I was absolutely exhausted. In the end, I had lost it all. Until you decide to make a change, nothing changes and apparently all that I had been through was not enough. I had gotten shaken up, but obviously not enough! Unfortunately, if you do not heal the wound, it repeats. It repeats until you decide to take the journey for yourself and heal the wound with intention.

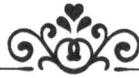

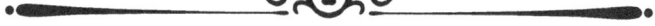

Chapter Seven
The Awakening

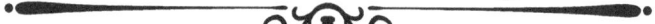

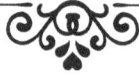

🙏 All the answers that you 🙏
are searching for are already
with in you. In order to find them
you must walk towards yourself.

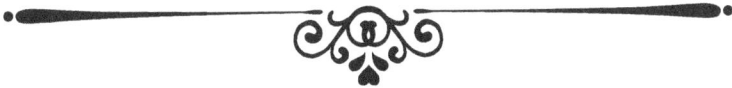

🙏 Rediscovering yourself will 🙏 be one of the most rewarding journeys that you will ever encounter. In order to do it you have to be willing to shed old layers of yourself that have outweighed their usefulness.

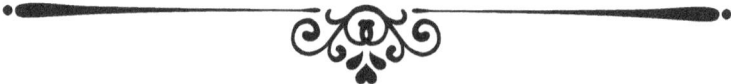

My awakening process began when I was in my mid-forties. It was memorable because it was prior to the relationship with Mr. "Ain't Got." In all actuality, the ball started in motion with the divorce of my ex-husband. It is the years in which all my puzzle pieces came together and my life started to make sense. Those were the years where I consciously decided to give up doing things my way and totally trust God. Those were the years in which I found myself and totally fell in love. However, it took the entire destruction of my life and a new construction of my soul for me to totally get the picture of my purpose.

The awakening is the process in which we begin to awaken from the deep sleep we were in from childhood conditioning. The sleep in which we were comfortable in our way of living, our choices, our pain. The sleep in which we were unwilling to change or even listen to something outside of our thought processes or conditioning. The awakening process can be gradual or it can be sudden. Oftentimes it is caused by something enormous happening on the outside of us to stimulate or awaken the inside. The process is intended to awaken us to our purpose. To make us aware that there are urgent changes that need to be made in certain areas of our lives. A purpose that we were either not seeing very clearly or a purpose that is being expanded.

I was so in love with Mr. "Ain't Got." In my eyes he could do no wrong. He had a gentle smile with a gentle touch. Who is Mr. "Ain't Got?" Mr. "Ain't Got" is a man that "AIN'T GOT" nothing. He "AIN'T

GOT" money, he "AIN'T GOT" a car, he "AIN'T GOT" a home, and he "AIN'T GOT" a job. Because we are so broken we decide to pursue the relationship anyway despite the red flags. After all the years of pain, betrayal, and foolishness, you would have thought that I would have learned my lesson and chose to do better. But nope!

I chose my own "AIN'T GOT"...yet again. We had known each other for years and he reentered my life when I was going through a difficult divorce. I would spend hours talking to him during the day, venting and releasing my deep intimate fears to him. I shared how I felt unloved, betrayed, and humiliated by my soon-to-be ex-husband. I was unhappy in the marriage and was at the very tail end of the divorce proceedings. Mr. "Ain't Got" came in like a thief in the night, an energy vampire looking to steal everything that I had. Or at least whatever I had left over from the divorce. He knew my secrets, my fears, and my insecurities and vowed to protect them and hold my hand throughout my divorce proceedings.

I had been in a relationship with Mr. "Ain't Got" about 10 years earlier, and it had not ended well back then. He had ghosted me, but through a twist of fate he ended up in the same state as me. With the divorce ending and the ex living in a different home, our relationship went to another level. Mr "Ain't Got" and I decided to exclusively date. Well, apparently, I was the only one exclusively dating.

He was aware of my boundaries, no cheating, fighting, devaluing, or mistreating my children. He agreed, giving me all the answers that

I ever desired and needed. I noticed that he was always seemingly unhappy and moody. Nothing in life would cheer him up. He would often say, "If you are happy, I am happy." I thought that this was fabulous until I later learned that he meant it in a way that was completely different from what I perceived it to be.

We spent time going on expensive trips at my expense. We traveled around looking at homes, looking at different states to restart our lives, and spent endless hours talking about our future. Later, those days went from spending time together to him disappearing for weeks at a time. He constantly found excuses to not spend time with me. He told me that he was going out of town for work, only to discover that he went out of town to spend time with another woman. It all came to a screeching halt when the side chick contacted me because she was upset that Mr. "Ain't Got" left her for another woman.

"How can he leave you if he is my man?" I thought to myself. At this point I had already decided to leave. It was then that I discovered that there were multiple women involved in the relationship.

He had spent our entire relationship stating that he despised infidelity and betrayal. I spent the entire relationship posting pictures proclaiming my love and intent for our relationship and he did the same thing. I was so proud to be with my "soulmate." I had multiple hospitalizations while we were together and was so impressed by his supportiveness. I had no clue that he was cheating with multiple women on the internet while he was sitting beside me while I was in the hospital bed. I confronted him about my concerns only to be disciplined by him via silent treatments, devaluing, and harsh words. One day prior to me speaking in Tampa at a Women's Empowerment event he exclaimed, "If you ever get on the stage, half of the people will walk out of the room!"

The next day arrived and I recall feeling very insecure as I walked up to the mic, those harsh words echoing in my mind. What if they do walk out? What if he is right? I walked up to the podium, shaking inside, grabbed the mic and spoke from heart. As I began to speak, my confidence returned. I knew that I could never remain with someone who had deliberately attempted to sabotage me just to make himself appear bigger. I realized then that he could not tolerate the attention being on me instead of him. As I suspected, everyone loved the speech and he walked out the back door. As fast as we fell together, we fell apart. Unfortunately, it was in the public eye. Eyes were watching, hoping for the demise of the relationship. He would often say that the only way that the relationship would be destroyed was if we allowed it to be destroyed. He told me everything that my soul needed to hear. I desired to be heard, understood, and seen as who I uniquely was as a person. We would take long drives, discussing how people did not understand us, the inner us. Mr. "Ain't Got" told me that he never loved anyone like me before and that I was perfect in his eyes. I loved him. He loved me. It was just an illusion.

One day, Mr. "Ain't Got" showed up at my house in a car. I often wondered where he got the car from because in reality, he "Ain't Got" nothing. He either caught the bus or I picked him up. He had never owned a car the entire relationship up until then. He told me that he got it from a friend's used car lot. He insisted that the friend recognized that he did not have a car and felt bad for him and told him to come and pick up any car that he wanted. I found that to be strange but Mr. "Ain't Got" insisted that the story was true, so I never asked about it again. He would pick me up and drive me to my doctor's appointments in that car on a regular basis. I remember asking him who paid the insurance on the car, and he told me that the car lot owner paid it. I never believed that story, but I could not prove that it was not true.

Every month, Mr. "Ain't Got" asked for money for something with the promise of giving it back. Every month, thousands of dollars left my hands never to be seen again. I was emotionally drained; I did not understand how he was unhappy. I was giving him the love that I thought that he needed.

The last straw with Mr. "Ain't Got" was when I was scheduled to have a major back surgery. The initial plan was to send me to a skilled rehabilitation center afterward to ensure that I would be safe upon arriving back home and learn how to regain my normal activities. The doctor knew that I would be unable to care for myself after the surgery and safely navigate around my home. I had a conversation with Mr. "Ain't Got" and he vowed to help me so that

I wouldn't have to go to rehab.

On my next scheduled appointment, I informed my doctor that I would not be needing inpatient rehabilitation services because I had full-time help at home. I was working in home health prior to my accident, so I was knowledgeable about all the post-operative equipment needed for this type of surgery. Looking forward to healing at home, I ordered all the equipment needed to assist with my rehab. On the morning of my surgery, Mr. "Ain't Got" drove me to the hospital but left during the actual surgery. He later returned to check on me but left after a few hours claiming that he had a cold. I ended up staying in the hospital for about a week and he never visited. He claimed it was due to his illness. I was in too much pain to even care.

On the day of my discharge from the hospital, I had to call around for hours to find Mr. "Ain't Got" so that he could pick me up from the hospital since he was my only ride. He dropped me off at home after we picked up the prescriptions from the pharmacy. He helped me get into the house, took off my shoes, and left. He claimed that he was too sick to stay and care for me. I remember struggling every day to make it to the bathroom. It literally took me hours to bathe and get dressed, but I was determined to make it. There were times that I went many days without eating because I could not make it down the stairs. I called Mr. "Ain't Got" and he either didn't answer or he said that he was busy. He returned to take me to my follow-up appointment and I tried talking to him about what was happening with us in the relationship.

"How did we get here? Why did you abandon me?"
He claimed that everything was fine and that we would be fine. When we returned to my home, I attempted again to have an in-depth conversation about the relationship. After all, I had forgiven him for everything that he had done. I was willing to move forward and just try and be happy.

"You want us to go there right now?" he asked with a smirk. I responded that I wanted to understand what was going on. "Things happen," he responded.

He got up and walked out the door and said that he would call me later. At that moment it felt as though my soul had left, too. It was just an illusion. Nothing that I knew to be true was true. After doing months of prior research, I finally concluded that my Mr. "Ain't Got" was a textbook narcissist! How in the world could I have fallen for this? I had cried for weeks, and it had never hurt so badly in my life. I begged God to remove the pain that I had. My heart was numb. How could anyone be this cruel and deceive people like this? I kept repeating the scenario in my mind. About six weeks later, I attempted to contact Mr. "Ain't Got" to get closure on the relationship. My mind was already made up and I knew that I was never going back but I wanted to look in the face of the man that broke my heart so intentionally. I met with him briefly knowing that I would never see him again, that our relationship would never be the same, and our friendship was questionable at best. About a week later after wrestling with my decision to walk away, I woke up out of a deep sleep.

"Walk away, now!" God said.

I had received the answer that I needed. I walked away and never looked back.

About three months later, it all came to a screeching halt when Mr. "Ain't Got's" side chick contacted me because she was upset that he left her for another woman. I knew that she was the female that he was sleeping with while we were together because people were telling me about various sightings and I saw internet posts of them together. The side chick told me everything. She told me that it was her car that he was driving while we were together and that she had given it to him because he needed a car. She described the clothes that she brought him while we were in a relationship and how they spent many nights together. She did not know that I was quietly taking notes during the entire relationship of his new clothes, shoes, etc. I knew that the clothes were a woman's touch, but they did not come from me. She told me about all his infidelities and how he took each of the women to the same places that we had gone. The interesting thing is that he even had the women begin to dress and look like me. The more she told me, the deeper the knife was pushed through my heart. Yes, I had walked away a few months earlier, but I didn't have concrete evidence of what he was doing. I had an intuition. This was my breaking point. I thought that he was a true friend and would never hurt me but he did to my core. I remember breaking down and crying harder than

I had ever cried probably in the last decade of my life. I hollered, I screamed, I grabbed my chest to catch my breath because at this point, I was hyperventilating. Then I ran for my life.

I ran for my past, I ran for my future, I ran for my freedom, my bondage, my survival. I ran until I could not run anymore but when I got up, I got up a new person. My awakening was now in full force. I told God that if he delivered me from this death grip of pain that I promise I would never return to my old ways. I promised God that I was willing to do whatever work it took to get to my place of healing, understanding, and peace. I did not know how I would do it or what it took, but I was determined that I was going to do it. I took a deep breath, gathered my thoughts, wiped my tears, and had an open conversation with God.

Me: "I've loved you all my life. I do not understand why I am here. I have worshiped you. I was a Proverbs: 31 wife. I am a good mother. I've never intentionally hurt anyone. I have been the best possible person that I could be. I have forgiven. I have been kind and patient. I don't understand how everything I've ever worked for has been snatched from me."

God: "Kellie, I have allowed you to go through this experience. I am taking you on a journey of healing. A journey to yourself."

Me: "I know, God. You are healing my body."

God: "No, I'm healing your soul. The reality is that you have not taken time out to deal with your past issues."

Me: "Yes, I have, God. I have dealt with my issues. I have conquered all my battles. I've walked away from people and moved on in life."

God: "No. You have been dealing, not healing. Yes, you have won the battles only to lose the war. The war that is raging inside of you. I allowed you to go through each experience for you to grow and learn lessons. You always had free will. Every time you called out to me I delivered you from the enemy's snare, but you kept returning to the battlefield. A different battle, but always the same war. This is the time that I need you to deal with all your past pain, so you can continue to minister to women and help awaken them to their purpose. However, I need you to minister to them through the lens of a healed woman."

Me: "But what will I do after the healing? I've been stripped of almost everything I have built. I'm exhausted."

God: "Have faith in me and you will come out like pure gold. You were placed in this life with a calling much bigger than you realize. Your gifts are still unfolding, but I need you to have faith. Follow the light!"

Me: "Ok, I will trust You with every breath in my body, but I cannot do it without You! I promise that if You hold my hand tightly during this process, I will never let go.

God: "Follow the light!"

After a long conversation with God, I came to a huge realization. It is time that we discontinue trying to minister to people from a place of brokenness without attempting to do the work on ourselves. It's time to stop pretending that we are perfect and misleading other souls, setting them up for failure and perfection. I knew what I had to do. I had to begin to make major changes in my life. I needed to heal some wounds. I needed to start from the beginning, the core of my pain. I was willing to run after God with everything that I had. I was willing to walk away from people, things, and my ego so that I would never repeat those cycles of pain again. I realized that I had placed my power in the hands of other people. I was allowing them to decide who I was and what I was going to tolerate and had allowed them to decide my levels of happiness and sadness. I decided to take my power back. To walk in my authenticity and live my truth. I decided that whenever I found ME, I would never leave her again.

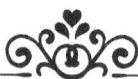

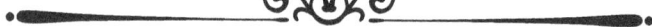

Chapter Eight
Acknowledging Your Wounds

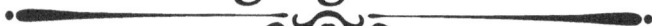

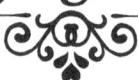

🙏 To heal you must be 🙏
willing to temporarily hurt.

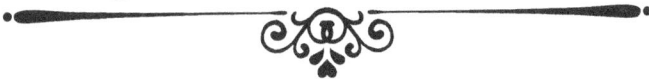

🙏 Healing begins the 🙏
moment you decide
to have an honest
conversation with self.

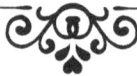

The moment that you decide to take accountability and acknowledge that you need to change the way that things are being done in your life is the moment that you begin to walk toward your true self and begin to heal. It is the day in which the momentum switches in a different direction. It has been said that the first step is always the hardest step. It is the step that is made sometimes with uncertainty, fear, or out of desperation for a change. It is a step that may have taken months or even years to decide on. Either way, it is not a step that can be skipped or made out of sequence.

The reality is that people believe healing is pretty and simple, but it is quite the opposite. Healing requires you to first ACKNOWLEDGE that you have some issues that require your immediate attention. That quite possibly these issues are contributing to your lack of growth or is at least stunting it to some degree.

Acknowledgment can look very ugly and its arduous work. It requires you to put a mirror in front of your face and confront every one of your wounds one by one. Acknowledging your wounds is going to require a pause in your life. A pause to deconstruct and reconstruct the new you. It is going to require that you take some time to sit in it and embrace all that you have in front of you. It requires an entire life analysis of your actions and reactions. It is going to require that you go to the basement of your soul and uncover some demons and all the buried wounds that have festered because they were left unattended for so long. The ones that you thought would either heal themselves or that you simply denied existed. The wounds that were easier to blame on others without taking accountability. It's going to require that you accept that perhaps you weren't as nice of a person as you thought or perhaps that failed relationship was partly or all of your fault, too.

It requires you to accept that you are flawed and you just do not fit the false narrative of perfection. The narrative that the world fed you as a child which was an absolute set up for failure. You cannot heal until you have first taken accountability and given yourself permission to heal. No one can do the hard work for you. Once you begin to take accountability your healing, power is activated within.

I remember that day so very clearly. It was the day that totally changed the trajectory of my life. The day that I decided to set myself free. On that chilly day in April, I stopped living my life the way other people thought that I should. It was the day that I was set free spiritually and mentally. I felt a huge weight lifted off me. In that same time, I consciously chose to raise my life to meet my expectations and not society's expectations. As you all know, I was in my late 40's before my huge awakening hit me like a lightning bolt. I had been on the quest for knowledge for about five years prior, but the awakening happened abruptly. I realized that I no longer wanted to be imprisoned in my mind. A self-imposed imprisonment. I realized that I needed answers that eluded me for my entire life. I needed answers to questions in which the answer made no sense. At least, in my life they did not make sense. I also looked at other people's lives and realized that their lives didn't make sense either. So how could they help me if they were running around in circles with their own life? My life had become a mental prison of insecurities and unnecessary stress. It temporarily destroyed and killed my dreams. I decided that I had to take that jump. It was a life-or-death situation.

The day that I accepted that it was okay to fail and that it was okay to not be perfect was the day I became the woman of my dreams. Not another person's dreams, but my own. I decided that I wanted to become a Queen Goddess and walk in my full power and purpose. I had accepted that I was fearfully and wonderfully made and that God's work had been and always will be amazing. I accepted that my life was my own to manage and to not give my power away at all. During this journey to self, I had to accept that I was human; a spirit having a human experience. A vital part of this human experience is acknowledging that I am and always will be the CEO of my life. I had been gifted with a pen. A pen with endless ink.

This pen is a gift given to all of us in the form of free will. It is the gift of choice. This pen can rewrite, strike through, and rearrange our lives as we see fit. With God, we co-write our own verses, chapters, and books. God is the author and we are the co-authors of our lives. So, what does all this mean? What does it look like? It means that you should and can make a particularly important decision to get back on track whenever you choose to. It is never too late to make upgrades, U-turns, or sharp rights on our journey. It is never too late to acknowledge our wounds and begin to make amendments to our stories.

When you take time out of your busy day and sit in stillness, you will begin to realize and recognize that out of all the pain that you have experienced, the common denominator is you. You begin to realize that you are walking around almost like a zombie on autopilot dealing with life through the lens of a broken person. Your steps become heavy as if you are walking in quicksand day after day on a the constant emotional rollercoaster of distress and feelings of unworthiness. Years of feeling defeat, pain, and unhappiness sit in your heart like unpacked luggage after a long trip: growing dust but much too overwhelming to unpack because thoughts of unpacking the pain leads to fear of losing control. Control of the emotions that you have bravely carried around, secretly afraid that someone would notice. Yet, you are praying that someone would stop and genuinely ask how you are doing. You are tired from carrying the weight for so long. Oftentimes, it's masked beneath weight issues, false identities, and facades.

Eventually after living so long in that mindset, you become your wounds and you unfortunately make friends with these wounds. The body has become accustomed to the weight. You walk around bent over, unsteady, slowed down, and heavy. However, you press through, never noticing that your body has become beaten down.

Lack of acknowledgement causes us to fight wars that weren't even assigned to our lives. We use our energy to blindly fight invisible wars that we aren't even going to win until we remove ourselves from it. Each time that you decide to use your energy to fight something that you have no power over, it weakens you! It weakens you because you are fighting an invisible enemy. An enemy in the form of a false narrative. The false narrative that you inherently lack the power within to make the changes needed. The false narrative that lies to you daily, waiting to strike you when you are experiencing even just a small level of doubt or apprehension about your worth. The invisible enemy that follows you around in the dark, waiting round the corner. Own your behavior, choices, and decisions! Do you want to be weakened by pain or empowered by strength?

One of the fears that has been verbalized to me on many occasions is the fear of change. Many individuals are afraid of what the journey will entail. They are worried about what people will think. People on the journey are also concerned about how the world will view them if they change or better themselves. These feelings are normal and can feel quite intimidating. All our lives we have lived, learned, and acted through the lens that was formed for us. The thought that there could be a different way of living can make many individuals feel quite uneasy. The thought that we do not have to remain in places in our lives to make others happy such as relationships, friendships, etc. can be quite frightening if that's all that we've ever known or seen. Toxic people teach you toxic ways.

They have nothing to compare it to because their role models were toxic as well. For example, if you grew up in a home where your mother was abused, the likelihood of you navigating to the same type of relationship is high, especially if your mother never left her abuser or received counseling. Not only did she need to receive counseling, but you should have received counseling as well to prepare you for adult relationships. Unfortunately, she probably did not give you counseling because she never received counseling when she saw her mother experience the same trauma.

Will people judge you or criticize you during this time? Yes, there is a great likelihood that they will judge you because what people do not understand; they judge. Will they understand your solitude or your thirst for knowledge for truth? Probably not. They will not understand it because they have not chosen to deal with their truths and will not know what it looks like to take this journey of acknowledgement and truth.

However, no matter what people think, say, or feel, your journey to self is a very personal one and should be taken only when you deem it necessary and when you are prepared to do the work intentionally and with purpose. This journey will require you to put yourself first and move some things to the back of your schedule that do not require your immediate attention. Let's be honest and transparent: some of these items can actually be delegated to someone else but because it's easier to remain busy than it is to sit still and deal with our junk, we decide to keep them on our to-do list. After all, it is much easier to fix someone else's problems than to accept that we too have problems that need fixing. Let us put ourselves first and begin to deal with the damages so that we can begin to live a much healthier, honest lifestyle.

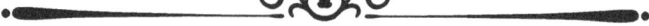

Chapter Nine
Damage of Unhealed Wounds

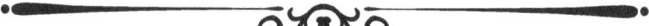

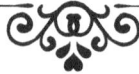

🙏 A person with an 🙏
unhealed wound is like
a neglected mansion.
How beautiful
it is... on the outside!

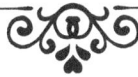

🙏 An unhealed wound 🙏
will never allow you to
discover who you are.
It keeps you imprisoned.

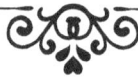

We, as spiritual beings, all share different stories, even though we may share the same wounds. The wounds may have been afflicted at different times of our lives, but they all have the same result. They have left us bleeding. We pull the knife out and slap a bandage on it in hopes that it will stop the bleeding. Yes, we may have to change the bandage several times in attempts to hasten the healing, but we never use antibiotics to deal with the infection. The antibiotic is truth. The truth is that we have not processed the pain. We were so afraid that if we took time out to process the pain, we may have to admit that we possibly failed, or the other person was victorious in hurting us. So, let us discuss a few of the damages to our souls that we may display. as a result of the damage that has occurred.

One of the scenarios that is often seen in individuals with unhealed Soul Wounds is that we run from relationship to relationship. We all know people who cannot be alone or have never been alone in their adult lives. We are afraid to face ourselves, and so we find ourselves in and out of relationships, looking to fill a void. We have no idea that it's actually an avoidance, but we know that we are searching for something. As wounded souls, we allow men or women to define who we are because of our insecurities of being alone. Oftentimes as children, exclusively women, we are taught to marry and find our "knight in shining armor" so that we can become "honest" women, as the old saying goes. We end up defining ourselves by our men and our relationships. We can become successful and achieve many things in life but people will still ask, "Where is your man?"

Subsequently, we go out our way to ensure that we always have a man on our arm. Not just a man, but any man, such as my Mr." Ain't Got." As long as he looks like a man and can keep us company, we are willing to embrace him as our own. Some of us are so broken that we are willing to be the side chick in the relationship as long as we are not alone in this world. We are willing to give of ourselves so freely so we can say that someone desires us. It is imperative that we stop giving the keys to our heart to people who are not even qualified enough to hold the keys to our car. We will not allow him to drive our car because of his reckless driving but we give him our heart without a second thought. The truth is that we have priced the value of the car to be much greater than the price of our heart and essence.

Unless you know who, you are, you should not ever invite anyone into your space. It is almost impossible to determine the right person or the right fit for you until you know exactly who you are. How can we show people how to love us if we have not first determined how we need to be loved? This type of reaction is a Soul Wound that looks to heal or deal with the lack of validation or value given to an Individual as a child.

Our inability to set boundaries or fragile boundaries is another deep, blistered Soul Wound. We all know people who are afraid to set boundaries. These are the individuals who are afraid to say no, or they say no and frequently change their mind. These are people who have very fluid boundaries. To heal these wounds, you must have very stringent boundaries because they are put in place to teach people how to treat you. People with fragile boundaries are generally people who stay in abusive relationships or friendships where infidelity, dishonesty, and devaluation are served regularly, just like dinner every night. We believe that our work is defined by other people's emotional reaction, unaware that we are not responsible for their emotional wellbeing but strictly ours alone. When you know your worth or your value, it teaches others how to treat you and love you. Constantly pouring into others with little or no regard for oneself is another result of damage caused by Soul Wounds. We show up for others who refuse to show up for us. For instance, we all know girlfriends that we call because we are feeling down and perhaps need a word of encouragement. We just want to tell them what is going on in our lives and discuss how we are feeling. However, they quickly direct the conversation towards themselves, how they feel, and how they are doing. They never stop and ask us how we are doing and so we feel as though the conversation was null and void because we never had the opportunity to express our feelings.

How about the girlfriend or family member who calls and dumps all of their stuff on us and never asks us how we're doing? These individuals eventually end the conversation feeling very refreshed, but we are left feeling very empty and very exhausted, like emotional vampires. There is an old saying that says that we must learn to put the oxygen on ourselves first in order to save others. We cannot pour from an empty cup because the reality is if you continue to pour from an empty cup, you are going to destroy yourself. The cup does not have to be full, but it has to be filled to some capacity. You are not truly able to love anyone at all in any capacity unless you have something to offer them.

This *Soul Wound* is definitely one of my favorites to discuss because we see this one more often than not. I call it the "Ole working 25 hours in a 24-hour day." This person is constantly busy from sunup to sundown. Almost like an octopus with eight legs; each leg is dipped into something different, constantly moving, and is never at rest. This is the mom of the year, the soccer mom, the chauffeur, the PTA president, choir director, fundraising queen/king, etc. This person is always busyfinding something to do and always finding someplace to be. They keep themselves busy so that it can distract them from their feelings. They are not interested in dealing with any of their wounds or situations. They feel as if they can ignore the problems, then they do not really exist. They are constantly pushing their issues to the side while telling themselves that they will deal with it later. However, later never comes. What is really happening is that person is trying to find value in something external such as their experiences or accomplishments instead of finding value internally. They cannot find value within because they have not stopped to even process what they've been through. Furthermore, they probably are not really interested in doing so. They know that if they really stop and find time to deal with all of those built-up Soul Wounds, they may fall apart.

Have you ever noticed a Negative Nelly? Yes, my Mr. "Ain't Got" was one, constantly angry at the world. They have a problem for every solution that you present to them. They enjoy being the victim. You must, at some point, remember that you are only a victim for a matter of time and then you are a volunteer. This is the person that's always gossiping about other people and their downfalls and putting other people down. They never reach out to elevate anybody else. These people do not like themselves, so in actuality they are projecting their negative energy onto you.

Always remember that people's behavior towards you is exactly how they feel about themselves. If this person is constantly angry, they're going to project anger towards you. They can't see the light, so they don't want you to see the light, either. It's probably something from their past that has triggered their behavior, so don't surrender to these emotions. Feel them, observe them, and respond, but do not react. In other words, when you get angry, do not attack anyone.

Don't make that phone call out of anger. Don't hit anyone. Sit in it and ask yourself where it came from and what you do with it. When you look within, you're going to see wounds and parts of you that have been affected, and that has never healed.

Another serious consequence of unhealed Soul Wounds that causes damage to our lives is our inability to advocate for ourselves. We become afraid to speak up even in the event where we are unsure or fearful. This is the prime type of victim that a predator is looking for. The predator or abuser seeks out children or even adults that they They believe they are damaged in certain areas, where they attack. For example, Mr. "Ain't Got" observed and listened to my abandonment wounds and that is where he stuck his dagger and injected his poison. A woman in an abusive relationship with abandonment wounds will allow a man to stay because she does not want to feel the pain of abandonment again. These men are predators. They use your love against you!

Now, what about an example in which people appear to be well put together yet they are broken? Let's briefly address this. You were invited to a special event weeks ago and you accepted the offer. The day has finally arrived and you carefully scrounge through your closet to pick the perfect outfit to compliment the theme of the event. After trying on various outfits, you decide on the one that compliments your curves. You then decide which pair of shoes would make the outfit pop and show off your awesome calves. Next, you pick your jewelry and your lingerie. After you shower, you decide to cover your body in some chocolate flavored shea butter to make your skin glisten. You spend an hour on your face, ensuring that you chose the makeup that's a bit costly so it will last throughout the night without frequent touch ups. You put on your outfit and carefully look yourself over in the mirror to make sure that no lingerie lines are showing and that you are satisfied with the entire look.

"Perfect, flawless, amazing," you say out loud. You get in the car ready to dance the night away.

You park your car and walk into the event. The women begin to stare you up and down as you walk into a room. No, you do not know them, but they cannot stand the sight of you. Not because you are disheveled or hideous looking, but because you are dressed like a queen. The icing on the cake is that as you begin to work the room, they continue to glare with envious eyes. You glance over yourself once again to see if perhaps there was a stain on your clothes. Then you pull your small, bedazzled compact mirror out of your Chanel purse to check to see if there is lipstick on your teeth. Nope. Everything is perfect. You return the mirror to your purse, shrug your shoulders, and proceed to enjoy your night.

The reality is they hate themselves because they hate that they are not you. We were so wounded as children that we believe we aren't good enough and that we don't look good enough, so we begin to walk with our heads down. Here is a newsflash: they are broken, too. They are broken because they believe that if they tell you that you look wonderful it will diminish who they are as queens. They are beautiful as well. All they must do is straighten their crowns and do the work on themselves.

People are so broken that they are hiding behind facades day and night, afraid to expose their true selves to the world. They believe that if the world sees their true selves that they will not like them. It is absolutely true that all of us have some not so pretty parts of ourselves but because of the brainwashing effect, we view other people as perfect. They are not perfect and indeed work ridiculously hard to put on the illusion of perfection. For instance, let us look at the models that we see on social media. You have no idea how long it takes for them to make up their faces. It takes hours and plenty of retakes to get the perfect picture. They are told where to stand as lighting is strategically placed and reflective mirrors are being used. It literally takes hours to create a photo to post. Even after all of this, the picture is airbrushed or edited for the perfect effect. What happens as a result? We become depressed and anxious to post the same type of pictures, not even considering that it is just an illusion.

Finally, I believe that the most damaging result of our Soul Wounds is the abandonment of our inner child. The child that wants so desperately to be loved, held, and adored. The child that used to laugh and see the world as nothing short of amazing. The child who trusted everyone and judged no one. The child who came into the world ready to make a difference before the world snatched the joy out of its eyes. The child that we walked away from because he/she was too hurt to carry into our adulthood. The child that awaits our return. The child who is beckoning us to return to self.

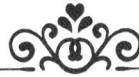

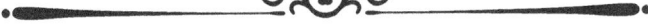

Chapter Ten
The Journey to Healing

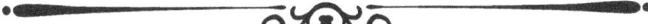

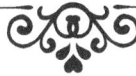

Hold your head up high so the jewels in your crown can shine as dazzling as you are.

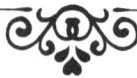

🙏 I promise to expose 🙏
my healed wounds
if it will help you
to heal yours..

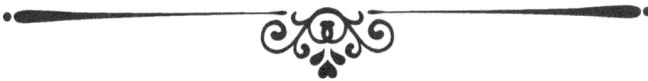

The journey to healing begins after the process of fully self-awakening and acknowledgment. After the awakening process, you become aware of the areas in your life that require healing and serious work. It begins the moment you decide that you no longer want to live according to the world's definition of you, but you want to know who you truly are deep down inside. Until you decide to do the work of healing you will continue to allow the world to dictate which direction to go, your worth, and your definition of love. It is almost as if you have lost your identity and you keep searching for it in the wrong place. The healing journey is one of intention. It's a journey that requires you to make a conscious decision to make changes in your life.

This part of the journey is overly critical and is going to require consistency, determination, and lots of focus. I suggest that you acquire a few items for the journey such as a journal, tissues, post-it notes, bubble baths, flowers, or anything that makes you feel beautiful. More importantly, I suggest a counselor, coach, or accountability partner. You need someone that holds you accountable and constantly supports and encourages you through this process. If you choose a friend, try and ensure that this person has already taken the journey and is currently transforming as well. Are you ready? We are about to dive deep and take the time to get transparent and naked with ourselves.

One of the first things that I suggest doing is to connect with your inner child, your God self. This can be done by getting rid of all the external titles that you have acquired; mother, sister, doctor, lawyer, etc. Remove the titles from yourself for just a few moments. These titles are not our whole story; they are just merely our external stories. You must be willing to let go of your old ideologies and way of thinking to go on a journey of transformation to your new self. Which means that this journey, once again, is very intentional. You must choose to get off the rollercoaster ride of dead ends. Your value does not come from the world's acceptance of you. We spend all our lives hiding behind our titles because we feel like they give us power. They give us recognition. We use these titles to hide that we are weeping inside. It is like a beautiful mansion that is dilapidated inside. You drive by and see a beautiful house with well-groomed landscaping, beautiful windows, and doors. It even has a wrap-around porch with a pool, but when you open the door...

The healing journey also includes disregarding your inner critic. That voice that says that you are not worthy, you aren't good enough, you aren't beautiful, you're not going to make it. Who do you think you are? You know, all those things that you talked yourself into in fear of changing your ways. You must get rid of all the false narratives that the world or your parents taught you. The people that you've trusted have taught you some things that just aren't true. They are false narratives. They often speak to you from their own positions of pain. It's not uncommon for them to inflict that pain onto you, knowingly or unknowingly. The negativity they speak into your life is not true. God formed you and knew you before you were born. The Bible states, "Before I formed you in the womb, I knew you before you were born, I set you apart" (Jeremiah 1:5). Then the world got to you and infected you with its poison. It was designed to prevent you from discovering who you are. The demonic force's plan is to speak to our spirit and convince us that we are not important and that we do not matter. You do matter and you are important. You are not who they say you are, you are who God says you are. God said that we are fearfully and wonderfully made (Psalms 139:14). Getting rid of the false narrative or that inner critic requires that you pause as soon as that negative thought arrives in your head. You must change that negative thought to something positive.

If there is something that you are told to do or asked to do on your job that you've never done before, don't tell yourself that you can't do it or you aren't qualified. Tell yourself that you can do it and that the only way you can learn how to do it is to experience it. The truth is that some things require experience and you can't learn it without actually performing it. The performance won't be perfect, but you are still going to learn from it. Never set yourself up to be perfect because perfection is an illusion, and we are not put on earth to be perfect. Strive for excellence instead. Remember that there is no such thing as failure if you have learned from the experience resulting in a positive outcome.

The solution to healing this negative thinking is to silence the voice. How do we do that? We do that by slowly reprogramming all the negative thinking. The first thing you will need to do is write down six things about yourself that you feel need improvement. That's also a part of the acknowledgement process that you have written down prior. Now, do the opposite by writing six affirmations. For instance, if you have low self-esteem, you are going to write, "I am worthy" on a post-it note. Do this for the remaining five affirmations and post them on your bathroom mirror or strategically around your home. In the morning when you brush your teeth, have a post-it note saying, "I am worthy." When you are driving to work, ensure that you have an affirmation in front of you on the steering wheel. Place it there the night before.

Another technique is using technology. Set your alarm clock to awaken you with a positive message to start your day. At the end of each day we are going to journal how the day went and set goals for the next day. Remember: it takes about 21 days to form a habit. The goal of this project is to deconstruct old ways and reconstruct new ways of thinking. We are transforming the mind.

Part of the healing journey is that you are going to go through a range of emotions, all of which may not be pleasant. I suggest that you use your journal to document all of these feelings. As you heal, layers of you will shed to allow for the new you. Allow yourself space to feel your emotions. In other words, if you feel negative emotions such as anger or depression, sit with those emotions. Surrender to those emotions, which means you feel them, observe them, but you don't react. The goal is to simply respond to them. If you're in a situation where you're angry, the goal isn't to lash out and take it out on someone else. The best response is to pause, sit, and feel that specific emotion and try to figure out where it came from.

Ask yourself what caused the anger because many times the situation that angered us is not the origin of our anger. You have to know why you're angry and what triggered your anger. You can also start by asking yourself questions about that emotion. For instance, you run into a female that provokes feelings of jealousy within you. Ask yourself why you feel jealous about this young lady? What is it about this person that makes me feel this way? What is it about me that triggers these feelings? It's going to be exceedingly difficult to start to confront those not so pretty parts about you, but it is a necessary part of the healing journey. This is probably going to be one of the most difficult parts of the process because as the emotions arise, it is best to take the time to deal with that specific emotion. As mentioned previously, the emotions will not always be positive, but it is quite possible that you must spend many days, possibly months, to effectively heal and deal with the root of your emotions.

Practicing gratitude is a great tool to use in the healing process. Focus on how far you have come, your personal achievements, and even the small steps in life. Practicing gratitude is one of the greatest things you can do because you are actually conditioning your mind down to the cellular level to be happy and appreciative.

With practice it will change your method of thinking negatively as a first response. It slowly changes your lens and what you see by deconstructing your old ways of thinking and reconstructing your thought process. Gratitude does not require you to travel the world to take in its glory. For you it could include walking around the neighborhood and taking in all the scenery.

One suggestion I have is to take a daily walk alone. What do you see? What do you smell? What do you hear? Once you return home, journal the answers to these questions. Being grateful for the birds that you see, the air that you feel, and the flowers that you smell. Gratitude is just the act of changing the way you look at things. Instead of looking at the cup half empty, you are going to begin to look at that cup half full. You are no longer going to focus on negative things even though they do exist. You're going to pull your focus away from any thought that pulls you down in a negative energy space. Remember that energy goes where your attention flows.

Forgive yourself for what you did not know because you were young and you had no idea the picture that they were painting for you was going to be poisonous. You had no idea that you could be any different than what you were instructed to be as a child. You had no idea that you had choices and that you had a voice. You didn't know that you didn't have to say yes, all the time. You had no idea that you were taught things by broken people. You had no idea who they were either. Your world was being conditioned when you were younger so do not continue to hold onto something that you did not create. However, as an adult you have a responsibility to make better choices. Do not continue to beat yourself up. Start to give yourself the unconditional love that was missed in your childhood.

Forgiving your parents or family members is also a crucial part of the healing journey. Forgive them for not parenting you in the way in which you needed to be parented. Remember, the likelihood that they were also wounded is high. It was like the blind educating the blind. It's time to have conversations with yourself that your parents never had with you. You know, those broken conversations. Conversations that your parents did not know how to have with you. Conversations that started and ended with, "Because I said so!" Conversations that left you confused and unheard. Yes, those conversations. It's okay to reparent yourself by giving yourself all the love that you deserve. Start over and start living your life the way that you've always desired. Always remember that perfection is impossible, but transformation is always possible.

Finally, and most importantly, start to trust your intuition. One of the greatest gifts that God gave us is our inner voice. That inner-God voice. The voice that will never lead you astray. The voice that we learned to not trust as children because the world made us second guess ourselves and how we felt. The voice that was not allowed to be expressed even when we felt danger or unsafe. You know, the times when we are forced to give Brother so-and-so a hug even though he would breathe heavily on our necks or squeeze us inappropriately. Remember, when we told an adult and they responded, "Oh that's Brother so and so, he is a Christian. He wouldn't do anything to you!" It's safe to trust that voice. You were right and the adults were speaking from their inability to deal with their own childhood encounters. Take your power back, trust your intuition, and allow it to lead your life. It was designed to be a light in darkness, to steer you away from danger, and bring you safely to the other side. You are no longer a powerless child; you are an adult with all capabilities to make your own decisions for your life. Yes, its difficult to change your mindset and come out of the past conditioning from your Soul Wounds. You were in a battle for your life, but you won! Now its time to continue your journey with all the knowledge that you have acquired along your path.

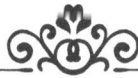

Chapter Eleven
Living in Wellness

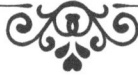

🙏 **There is freedom on the other side of pain**

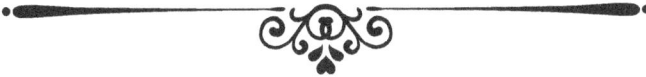

🙏 Your purpose is hidden 🙏
in your journey to self.

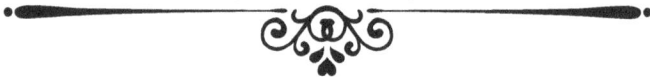

Healing from your Soul Wounds is not something that is going to happen overnight. It is going to be a lifelong process depending on where you are in your life cycle. Choosing to be free and independent from your past pain and wounds will be one of the best decisions that you will ever make. The best part of the journey is that you will find your purpose after all the smoke clears. You will begin to realize the significance of letting go and surrendering to the evolution of the new you. Though the final results will not be immediate, you will begin to realize that after you have dug into the depths of your soul and healed the wound, your vision will become clearer and the noise won't be as loud. You will begin to hear the voice of God clearer and you will make better choices in your life. You will begin to live in a wellness state, a state of tranquility. You will notice that all the puzzle pieces will begin to make sense. Then you will understand that the pain was all a part of a greater lesson if you chose to not give up. The decision to move on and never look back is such a great step towards living your best life. There is truly freedom on the other side of pain.

Living in wellness may look completely different than you imagined. Your eyes are going to open to all the spiritual aspects of the world. You will begin to recognize good vs. evil and spiritual vs. carnal. The Bible states that, "For our struggle is not against flesh and blood, but against the rulers, against the authorities. Against the powers of the dark world and against spiritual forces of evil in heavenly realms" (Ephesians 6:12). Once you have awakened you will begin to pursue things of the spirit and things of the flesh will be less appealing. The foods that you used to like will change; your body will now decide to feed your spirit. The men that you are accustomed to dating will change. You will no longer desire to date an individual who does not vibrate where you are currently vibrating. The Bible states in 2 Corinthians 6:14, "Do not be unequally yoked with unbelievers." The reason for this is that the unbeliever will begin to intoxicate your soul with things of the world. They will cause you to focus on the flesh instead of the spirit. This behavior will lead you back to where you were before the journey. It is best to socialize with people who have the same goal of self-healing and evolution. It's also beneficial to evaluate all of your friends to see where they need to be repositioned, if at all, in your life. Once you have started on this journey you will find that some of the people in your life have outweighed their usefulness and that is okay. Perhaps in due time they will fit in your life in their proper place but for now it's imperative that you continue to focus on a healthy life journey.

As you transform and heal, so will your thinking. You are going to start to realize that all the things that you thought were true were false narratives designed to destroy your journey of self-discovery. Now that you have transformed your belief systems, do not be surprised when you experience a renewed sense of freedom. That freedom will come when you decide that you are going to live in authenticity. Authenticity is when you decide that the world will no longer dictate what works for you and you begin to trust your inner guidance. You begin to embrace everything that is different about you and what makes you unique. You will understand that you were never designed to fit in but to stand out. However, there will be steps that you may want to consider in order to maintain your newfound wellness. We all know that after a significant transformation process it is going to take hard work to maintain it. Let's discuss a few techniques that I have found work if used consistently.

The first suggestion that I have is to continue to embrace spiritual direction. My guidance is the Bible. The Bible states in Ephesians 6:13, "Therefore put on the full armor of God, so that when the day of evil comes, you may be able to stand your ground, and after you have done everything to stand."

If your choice is not the Bible, try to embrace some divine spiritual guidance that teaches you how to continue to walk and commune with God Almighty. Be mindful not to get caught up in negative practices, which may be tempting due to pressure from the outside world. The Bible warns us of false prophets that come to you in sheep's clothing, but inwardly, they are ravening wolves (Matthew 7:15-20). Because the war on this earth is good vs. evil, the enemy's job is to distract along the journey. The goal is for you to become or remain so distracted that you can't discover yourself. If you discover yourself, you will discover your purpose. So, be aware of individuals who are seeking to give you false guidance along this journey of wellness and discovering you. This part of the journey is going to require constant awareness. Begin to pay attention to everything that's around you.

"Do not believe every spirit but test the spirits to see whether they are from God, because many false prophets have gone out into the world" (1 John 4:1).

Pay attention to the people that you're around, to the words that people speak to you. You will also notice that even though you have chosen the path to truth, it does not mean that others are also doing the work on themselves, so don't be quick to judge. Try not to judge at all if possible. It's simply where they are in their life journey. They are still unconscious and they will not understand the path that you're taking. There will be times when people won't understand where you are in life because you've changed and you no longer want to be a part of the same crowd. The things that people do not understand tend to make them very uncomfortable.

The reality is that many people are walking around wounded and have not chosen to take the journey of self-healing. Many have not even acknowledged that they are wounded. They have decided that it is much easier to remain in the state that they are in rather than to deal with the deeply rooted pain. The result is lack of self-awareness. People walking around who have no idea who they are or who they were formed to be by the divine creator. Job 32:8 states that there is a spirit in man. A spirit in man simply means that we are spirits having a human experience. These wounded individuals have not reconnected with God spiritually and are continuing to follow their fleshly desires.

Once you have started on your path you will begin to notice that people will become jealous or envious of your changes. You will indirectly shine a light on their insecurities and wounds. Though the journey is not intended to directly affect others, it will cause a mirror to be placed directly in their face. So be very cognizant of others around you who may intentionally mislead you back to old behaviors. These people will also continue to speak to you from their broken places. Remember that you have chosen the path for your life in this moment and they are still searching for direction. As a result, they may continue to speak negatively to you. Don't take it personally; it's all a part of the bigger picture of deciding who is in your soul tribe.

As I mentioned before, journaling is also a great technique to use throughout your healing process. Even after the healing process is done, journaling allows you to put your feelings on paper so that you can go back and compare and contrast where you were and where you are now. The journal entries will demonstrate to you how far you've come and the things that you need to perform differently. The journal will allow you to see your goals at a glance. It will encourage you when you can't find encouragement anywhere else. Once you see how far you've come you will begin to understand that the goal is within reach.

There will be times when there aren't many encouraging people around you on this journey. So, your best cheerleader will be yourself. My suggestion is to keep a journal by your bedside at night and perhaps write down your goals for tomorrow. Also write down your daily accomplishments no matter how small. Small accomplishments lead to great goals,

Meditation is also a suggestion. Mediation allows you to continue to go within and deal with your emotions. It allows you to find your power and connect with the divine God within you. It also allows you to clear your mind of all the negative thoughts that may have crept in your mind early in the morning or late in the evening. Whatever time you choose to meditate isn't as important as the outcome of the mediation itself. The ultimate purpose is to remind you that you are strong and powerful. Learn to talk to yourself in a beautiful way. Learn to encourage yourself. Learn to remind yourself that you are powerful beyond belief.

Learn to adopt mantras. A mantra is a positive statement or slogan that you will repeat out loud every day. The purpose of the mantra is to inspire and motivate you to be your best self. It also sends positive energy out into the world and gets you accustomed to having a positive mindset. One of the exercises that I previously suggested is writing mantras on post-it notes and stick them everywhere throughout your home. Post one by your bed to see first thing in the morning. Post one in the bathroom by your mirror. Post one by the stove. Ensure that each post-it note says something different. Read them out loud when you see them. Try to read each of them several times a day. Also set your electronic devices to awaken you to a positive message to start your day. These exercises not only motivate you, but they raise your vibrational energy.

Raising your vibration is a vital part of your healing journey. There are many ways in which you can raise your vibration. You can raise your vibration by listening to music. When you choose music, try to choose music that has inspirational lyrics or songs that are extremely upbeat. You can raise your vibration through dance or just by focusing on anything positive. Continuously feed your soul positive information. This means that you may have to turn off the news or limit your social media interactions. You may even decide to screen phone calls and allow them to go to your voicemail. It does not matter if you choose to do all of the above or just a select few as long as you make an honest effort to find your place of peace.

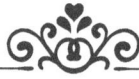

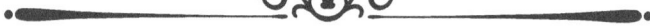

Chapter Twelve
Your Eyes Through the New You

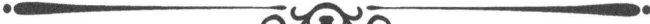

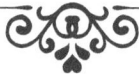

🙏 Wrapped within your 🙏
pain is your purpose.
You just have to open it.

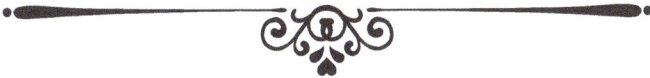

🙏 Your Purpose is buried 🙏
In Knowledge of Self.

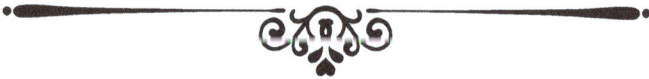

Your brokenness is where you find your anointing. For reconstruction to properly occur, there must be a deconstruction of the foundation. Deconstruction to the human eye is never beautiful. It occurs with bittersweet memories and sometimes some uncertainty. However, it is necessary.

Sometimes, you must sit in it, experience it, and embrace it. See it through in its entirety. Yes, it's going to hurt, you are going to cry, you may even get angry and punch a wall. But there is no way over it, under it, or around it. You had to take that bandage off.

Because of your healing, your next generation will be healed and delivered from those strongholds. The enemy knows that if he can keep you stuck in a place of depression, oppression, suicide, and rejection, your gifts will never be released because you will never trust yourself. You will never believe in yourself. You will second guess every decision that you make. In your weakness is where God's strength will be found.

All the wounds that you have conquered, all the pain that you have endured, was not designed to break you but to make you. It was designed to help you discover your purpose, to truly see yourself through an entirely different set of lenses. Lenses that are no longer clouded with pain and despair, but clear with hope and joy. It was designed to set you onto your path of freedom. Freedom from the world and freedom from the old you. No, God never left you and God was not punishing you. God was molding you into the person that you are today. No matter what situation you were born into, you were and will always be so very loved. Your existence is not predicated on the opinions or the validation of others. You were divinely orchestrated and created to be in this moment, at this time, in this space.

One day you are going to sit back and realize that all the loneliness that you endured was to help you see that you had the whole world in front of you. That it was not the ending, but it was simply a pause. A pause in your life where God needed to do some work on you. A pause for you to self-reflect and redirect.

During this pause you will begin to pursue that passion that you always had hidden away in the back of your mind. You will begin to understand the reason why you took that specific path was to make others happy and that you were never happy. That your desire to please others was so strong that you did it anyway, putting your dream on hold because someone swayed you away from it as a child. You will begin to pursue the things that you enjoy and realize that you have finally unwrapped your purpose, your gift. You will begin to confidently walk in your newfound purpose, realizing that you now feel free. People will notice that you are happier, less stressed, and that the gift you refused to use is now changing so many lives.

What God desired to help you realize is that when it appeared that you were never going to make it, He forever held your hand and caressed your forehead. Through all the tears, the fears, and all the lonely nights, He never left your side. Even in the darkness, that tiny flicker of light in your distant view was God. Even though it felt as though you were constantly surrounded by darkness and could not find a door or an exit sign, know that God was standing there beckoning you to come forward.

Soul Wounds: a journey wrapped in pain, filled with salty tears. You have accepted that it was never about being perfect but about experiencing life. The lessons are in the wounding experiences. Regardless of how the wound was inflicted, you are not it , and it is not you. You have overcome, you have discovered YOU. You have taken a journey back to yourself. You have discovered that to be uniquely you, you must have the audacity to live outside of the box and draw outside of the lines. As you place the last puzzle piece in position you will soon discover that it fits perfectly. You glance closely at the final picture with tears in your eyes.

You stare at the puzzle in awe as it slowly sinks in. It is a woman walking towards her inner child holding the final piece to the healing journey. The missing piece was you. You have been healed. You have finally rescued her. She is free.

🙏 Epilogue 🙏

In February, after petitioning the state for my adoption records, a social worker returned my call.

"According to these records, your mother fought extremely hard to keep you. She went all the way to the highest court to stop the adoption and apparently the state ruled against her. I'm not sure what you have heard, but your mother fought exceptionally hard for you. She wanted you."

I remember hanging up the phone and crying for hours. Those were the words that I have always wanted to hear. I WAS FREE. MY MOTHER WANTED ME. My biological father and mother had died years ago and left me with so many questions and a continued sense of abandonment. She had spoken from her grave. On that day I was set free, I was loved.

Today, I trust myself. No more allowing people to write my story. No more walking in fear. I was tired of living the way that I have been living. Afraid to draw outside of the boxes, afraid to choose the wrong color. I saw the picture, but my fears drew it differently because the world told me that it should look a certain way. That was not my experience. My experience was colorful and bold, filled with excitement and love. I was determined to paint that into a picture. Though it was a tough journey, I cried the entire time that I wrote this book. With the transparency came the memories of wounds that I never knew that I had. Memories started to return, and pain started to resurface. The tears were a relief because I knew that with each one there would be newfound hope. I knew that I was shedding layers of the old me and welcoming the new me.

As far as Mr. "Ain't Got?" Well, he still "Ain't Got" nothing, but I have never dated him or another one like him since. As a result of me healing my Soul Wounds, I've discovered my purpose. I now coach and mentor women who had their own "Ain't Got" experiences. Guess what? One of their "Ain't Gots" happens to be my ex! Yes, my ex. God has a sense of humor!

🙏 "The Light" 🙏

A child sits alone in an empty cold dark room, crying.

"Where has everyone gone?" she thinks. "I'm lonely and afraid." She pulls her doll closer and reaches over to grab her book. A small puzzle piece falls to the floor as she opens the book. "Oh, there you are. I've been looking for you for a long time!"

Tears begin to well up in her eyes at the thought of having to play with her toys alone another day. She places the tiny puzzle piece in her top pocket and continues to weep. She looks up through tear-soaked eyes and peers at the familiar bright light flickering in the far distance. The light has been the one constant thing in her life, always watching her in the distance. It illuminates her path when she feels lost and embraces her when she is sad. But today, it is different. Today, it beacons her to come.

She stands up, wipe her face on her tear-stained shirt, and begins to walk slowly toward the light. She is nervous, unsure of what lies ahead in her journey. She glances down and see a puzzle piece on the hardwood floor. She picks it up and it reads, "Rejection." She places it in her right pocket and continues along her path. The light beacons her again, and she moves slowly towards it. Along her path, she notices another puzzle piece, then two. She picks one up; it reads, "Humiliation." She picks up the other; it reads, "Betrayal. She places them both in her left pocket.

As she gets closer, she feels the familiar warmth of the light on her face. She recognizes its energy but is still unable to make out the form. As her confidence increases, she reaches down and picks up the remaining puzzle pieces: "Injustice," and "Abandonment," and holds them in her left hand. As she gets closer, she notices that the light has brightened and has taken on form. The child looks at the form and recognizes that the beautiful soul has missing pieces. It appeared to be a woman who was wounded, leaving holes in her soul.

Remembering the puzzle pieces that she found along her journey, the little girl quickly handed the woman the pieces that she was holding in her left hand.

"Perfect fit!" the little girl cried out. She reaches into her pockets and hands the woman the remaining puzzle piece that she had collected one by one. With each piece placed, the woman's soul begins to illuminate brighter, and her wounds began to disappear.

"How beautiful!" the little girl exclaims as she jumps up and down. "Can you stay and play with me? I'm so lonely."
"I was always here; I was Your Light. I'm back. I had to go away in

the distance to protect you, but I'm here now. I took the pain so that you wouldn't have to feel it." The woman lovingly states.

The little girl looks closely at the woman and notices that one area of the woman's soul nearest to her heart was a bit dimmer than the rest. It was missing a minuscule puzzle piece.

The little girl suddenly remembers the puzzle piece that she had carried her entire life. She reaches into her top pocket and grabs the tiny puzzle piece and it immediately starts to illuminate.

The woman reaches towards the child as the child hands her something that she is holding in her right hand. It is the final missing puzzle piece. The woman reads the piece aloud.

"LOVE."
The woman slowly places the last puzzle piece by her heart.

"Now you are healed!" the child squeals. As soon as the final piece was placed, the woman's entire soul illuminates, showing her entire face. She was whole! Chipped, but not broken.

The child gasps as she stares into the woman's face. She recognizes the face. She recognizes the energy. She recognizes the soul.

And in that very second, she recognizes that the woman she is looking at is HERSELF. The child realizes that the bright light was her the entire time. She has rediscovered herself!

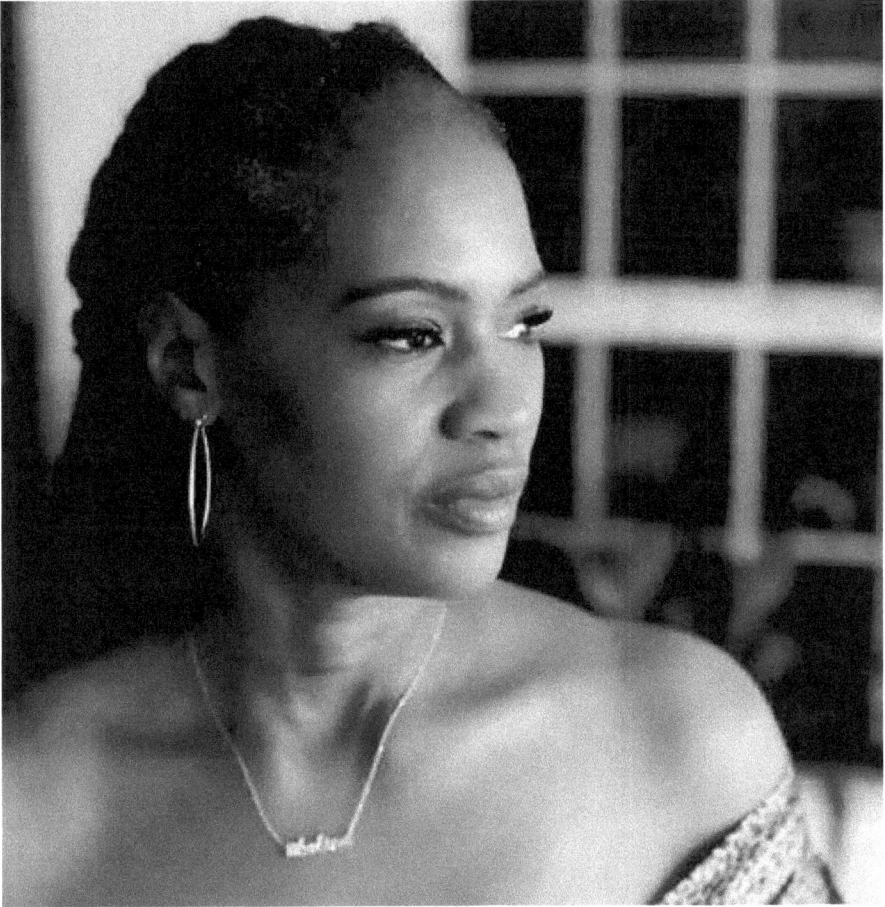

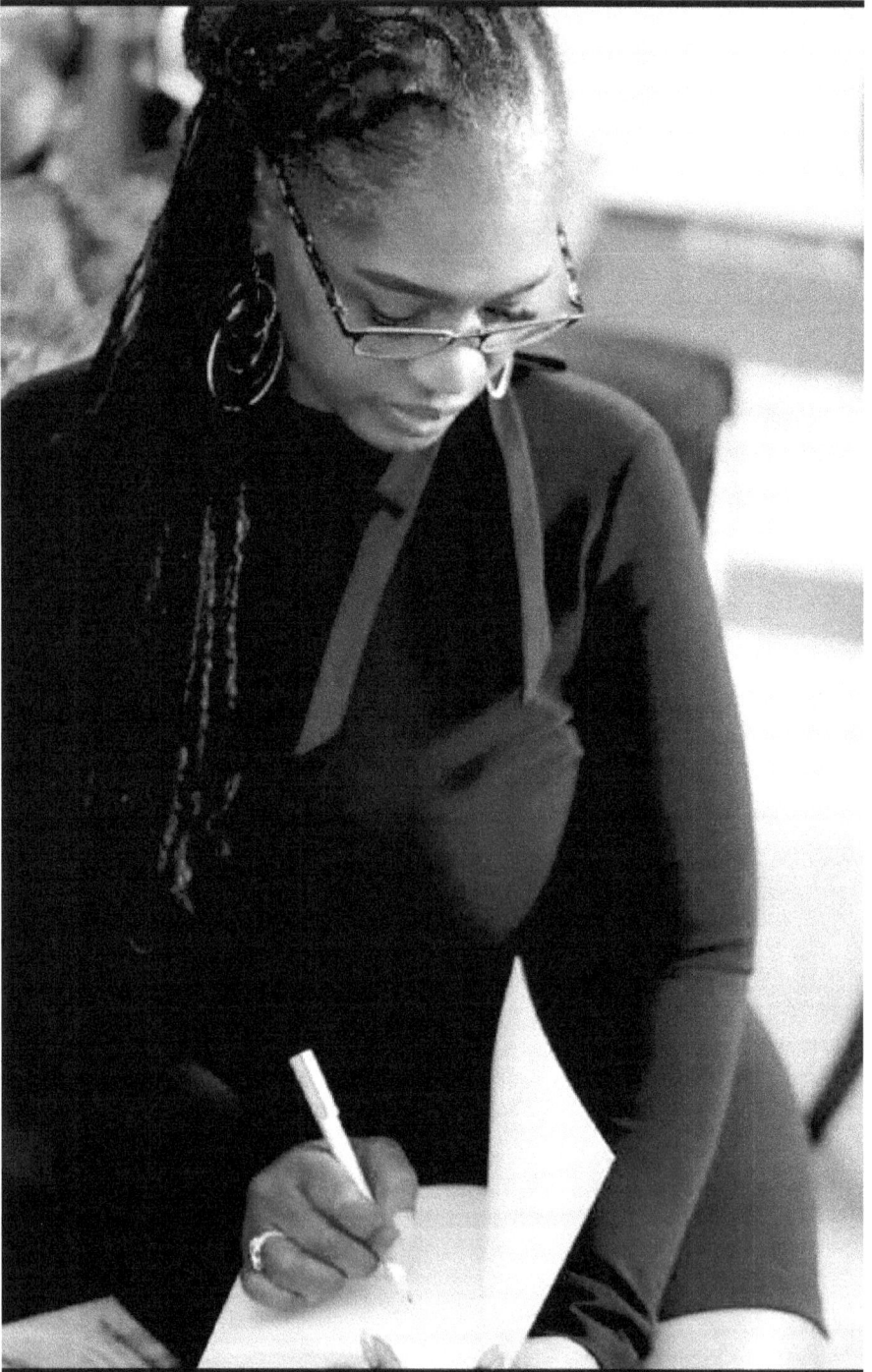

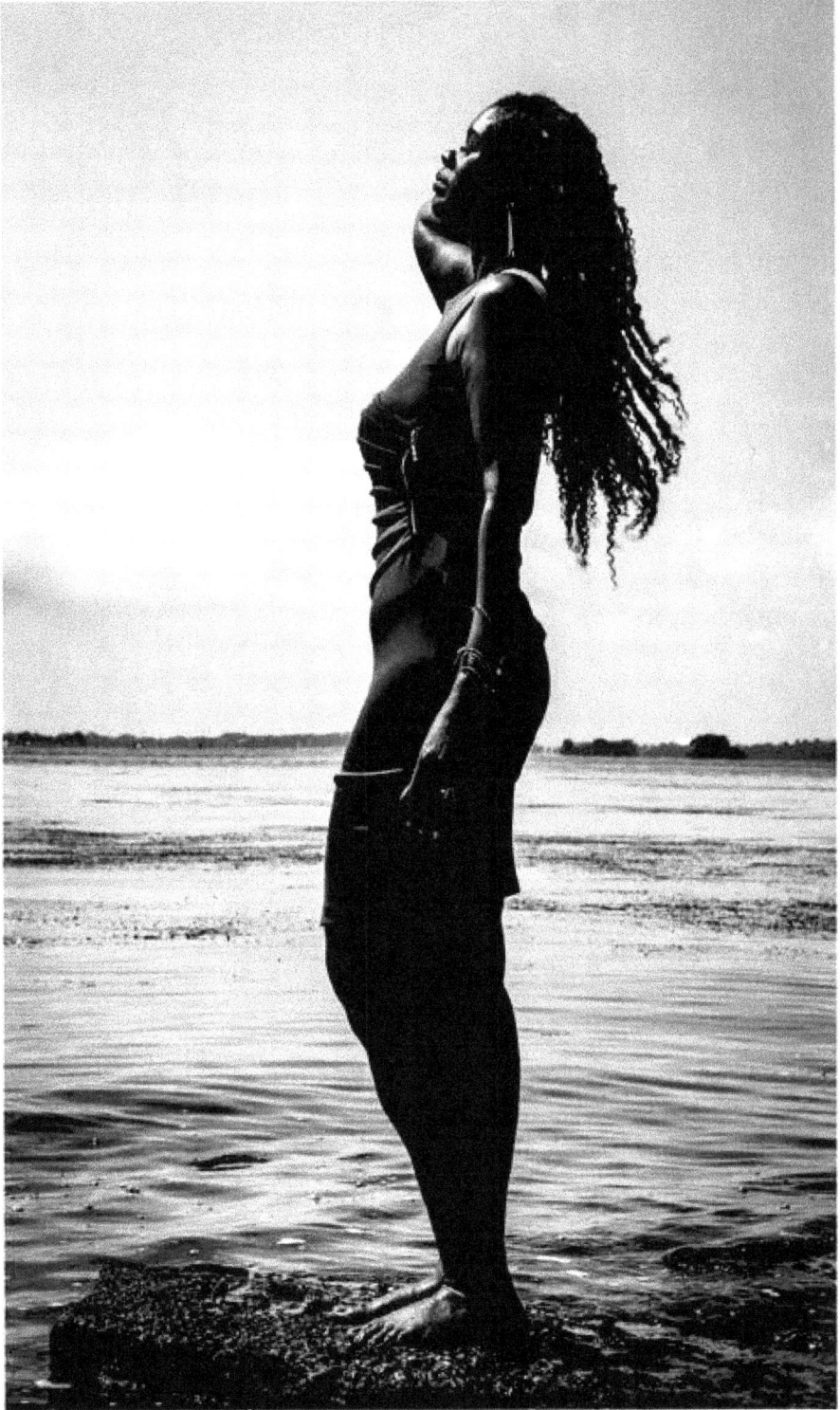

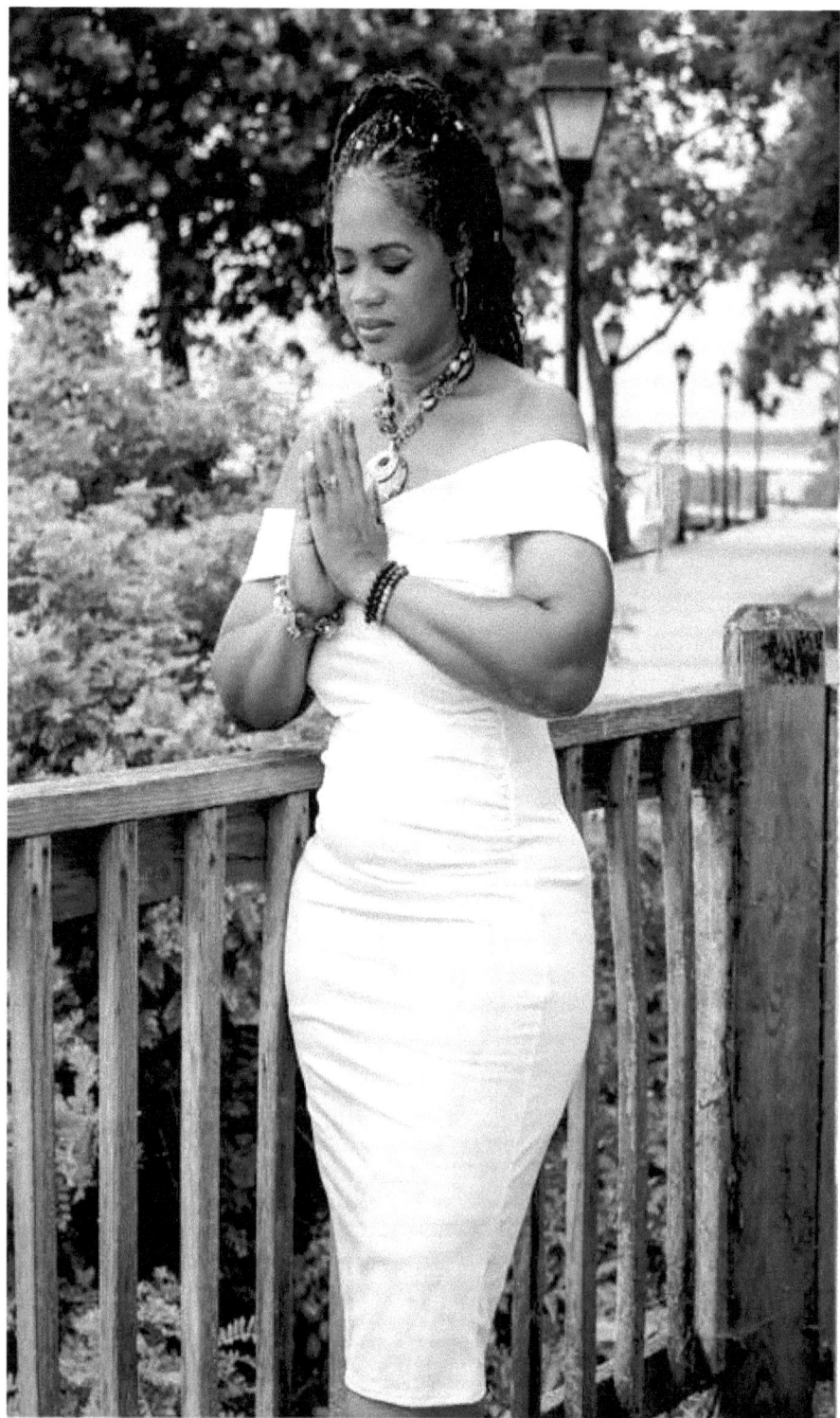

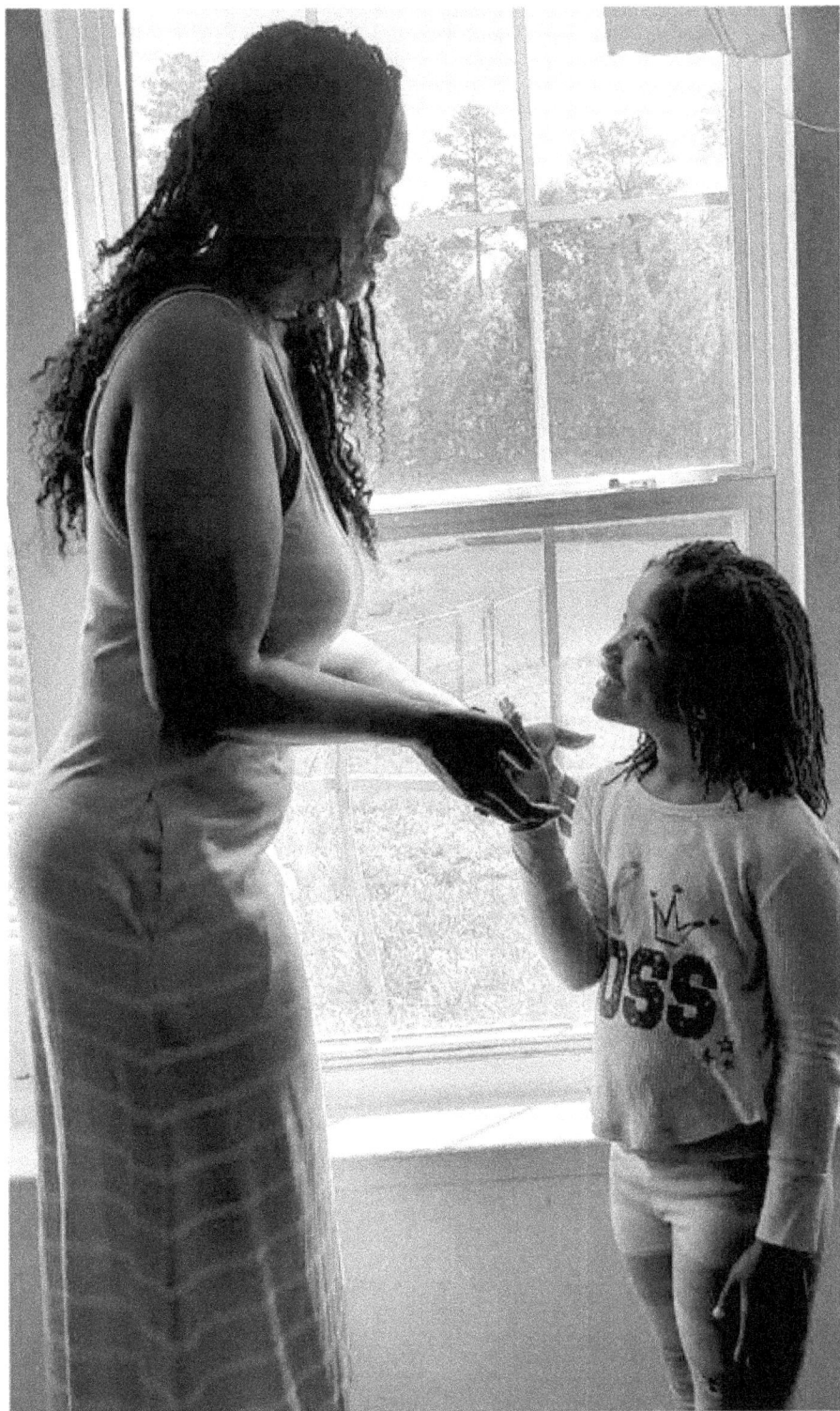

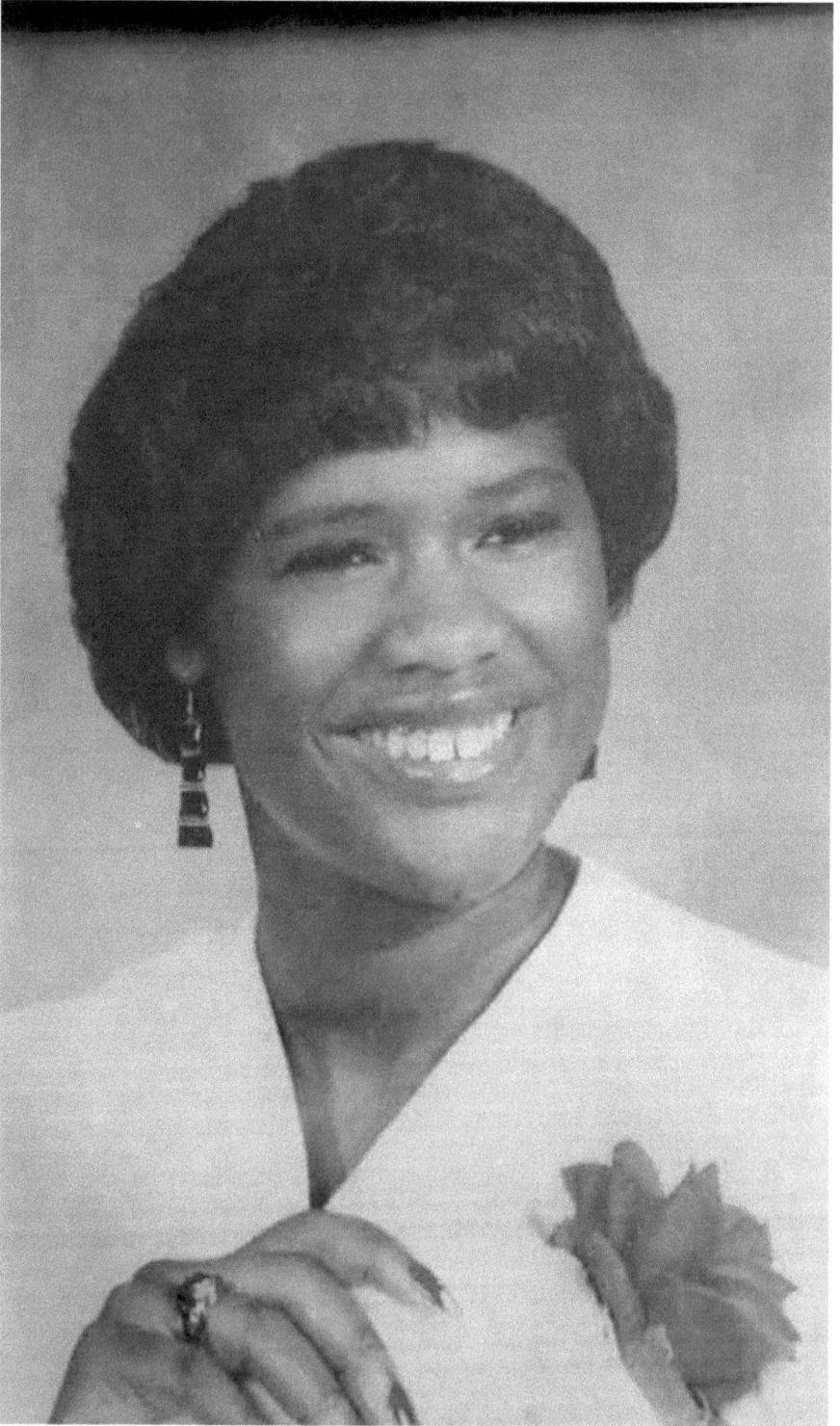

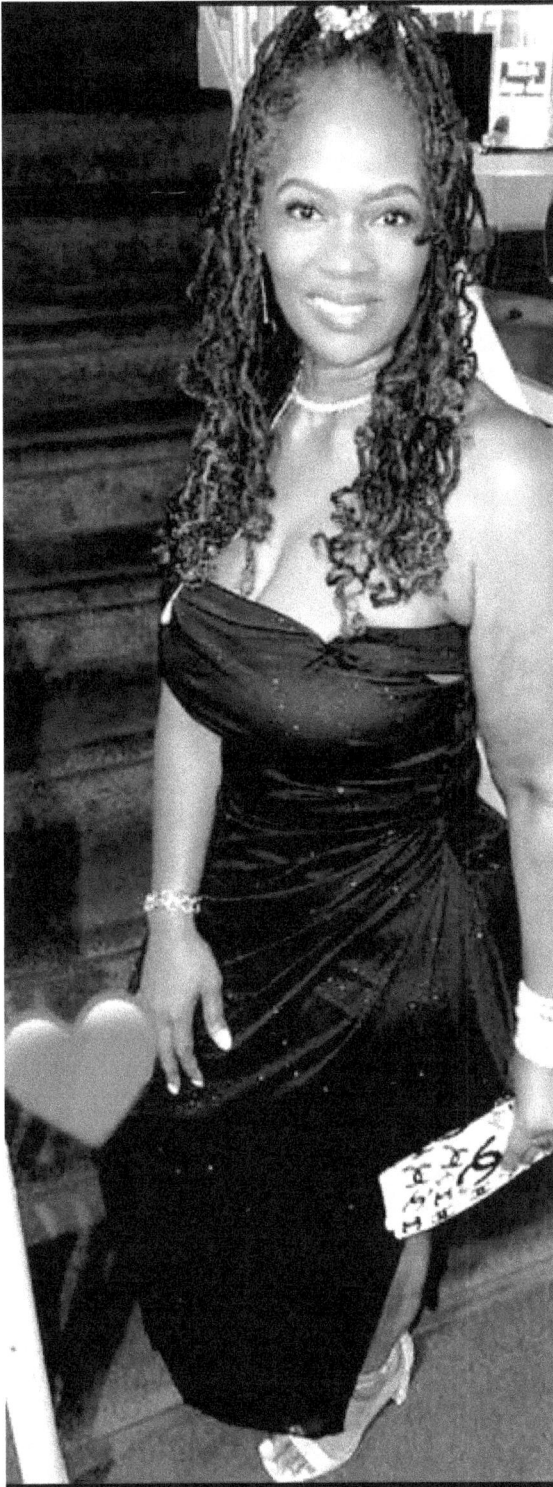

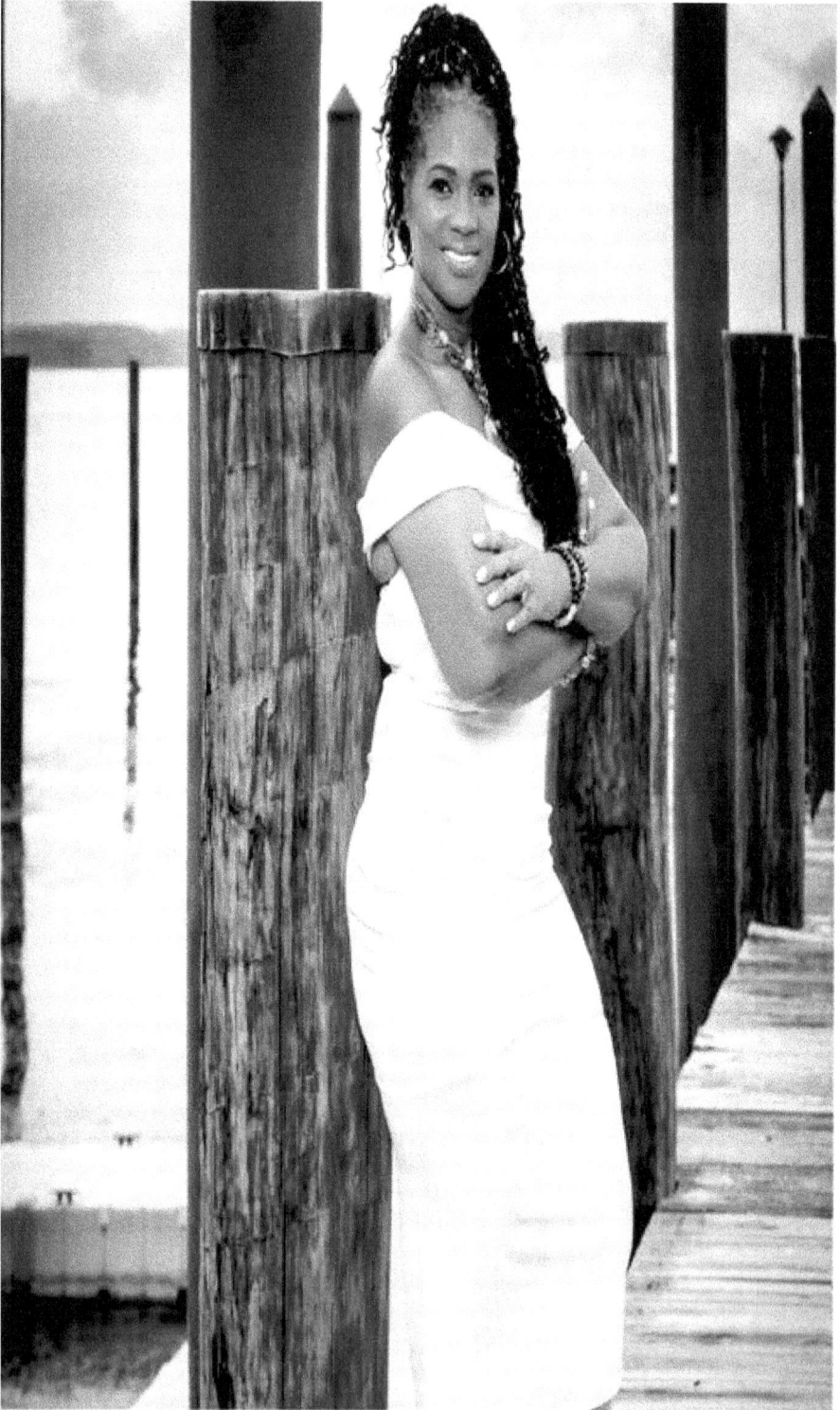

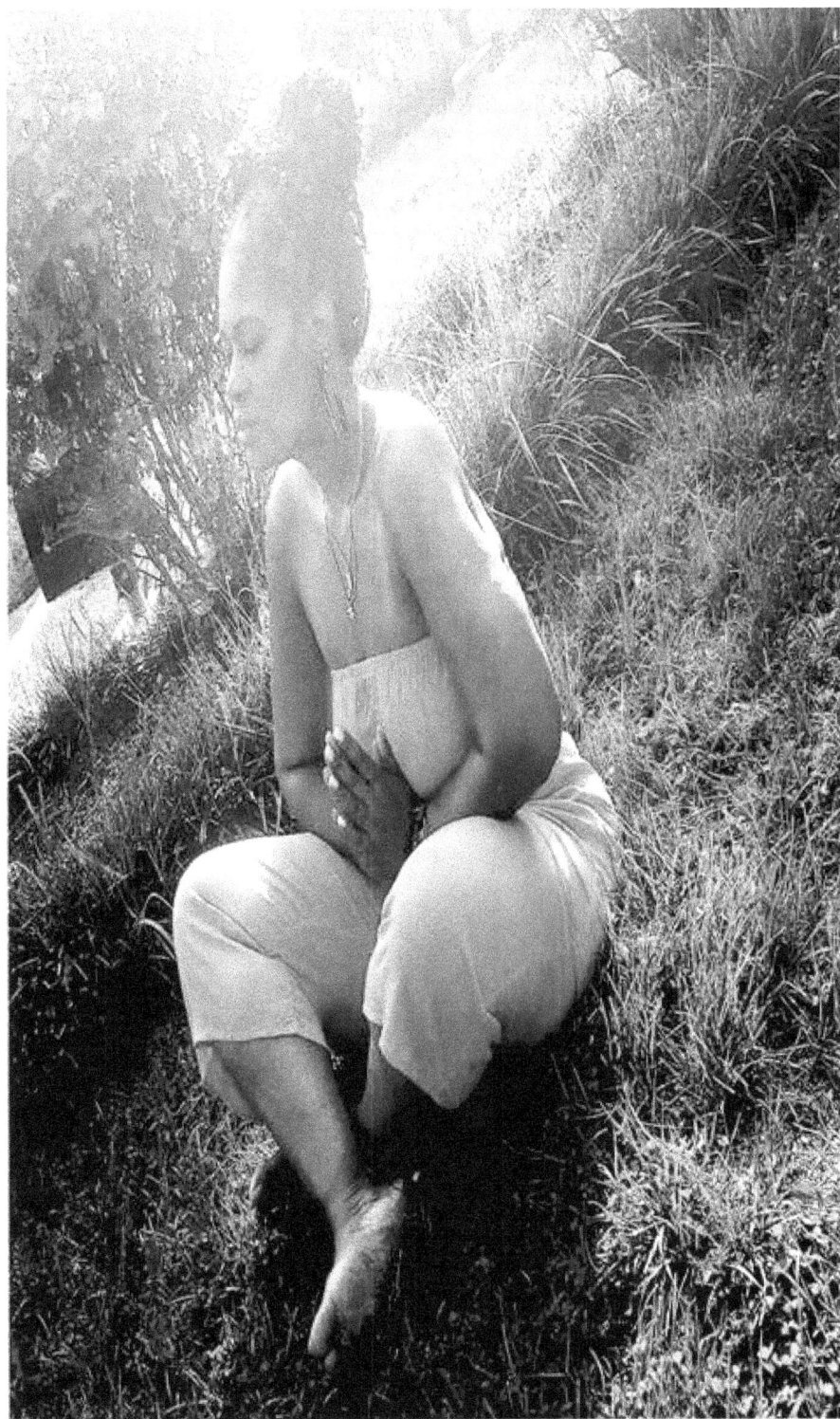

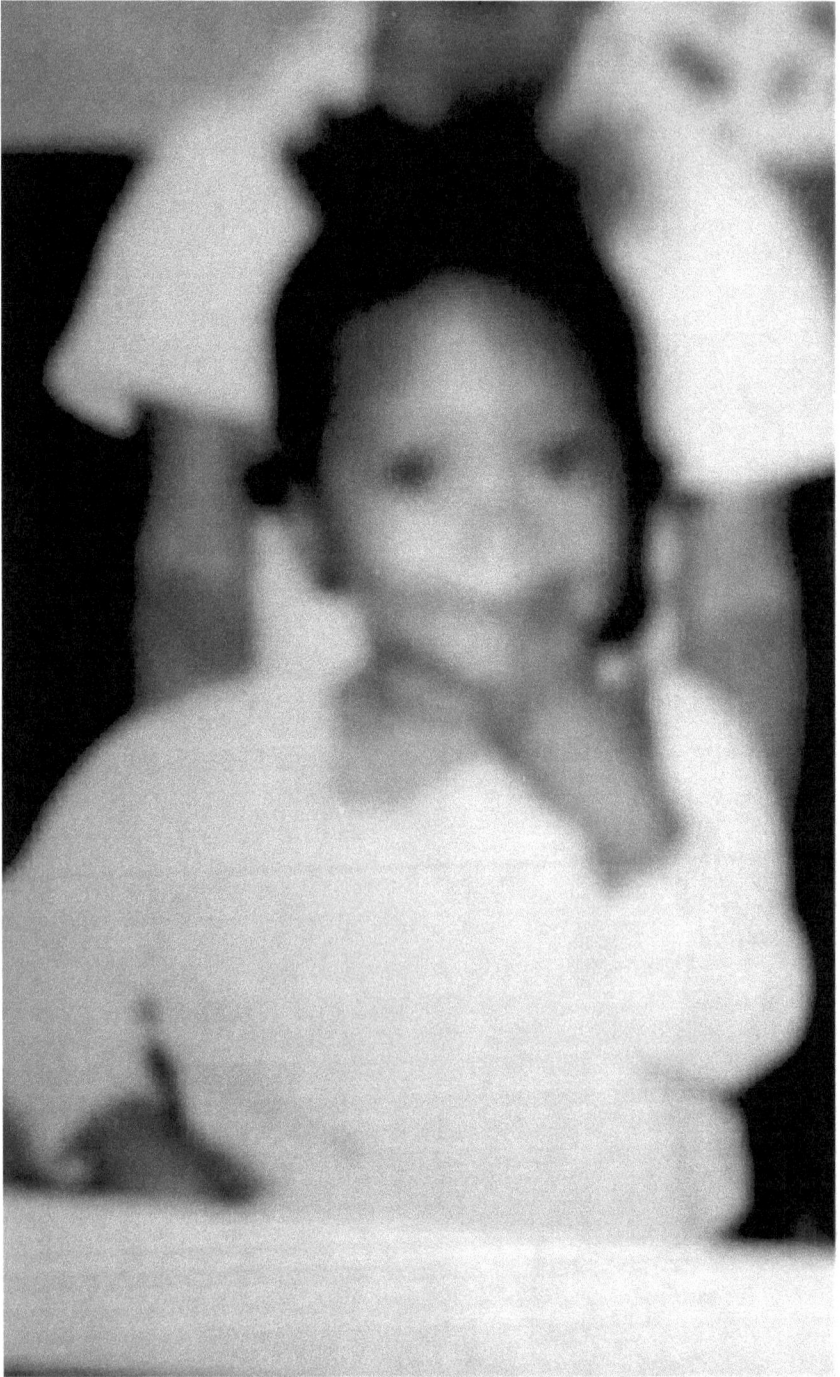
My only childhood photo

Congratulations.
nana for making
that book.

anyway can i
come over your
house someday.

from
Sterling

To Nana

Good Job on

making your

own best.

I love you.

—Makai

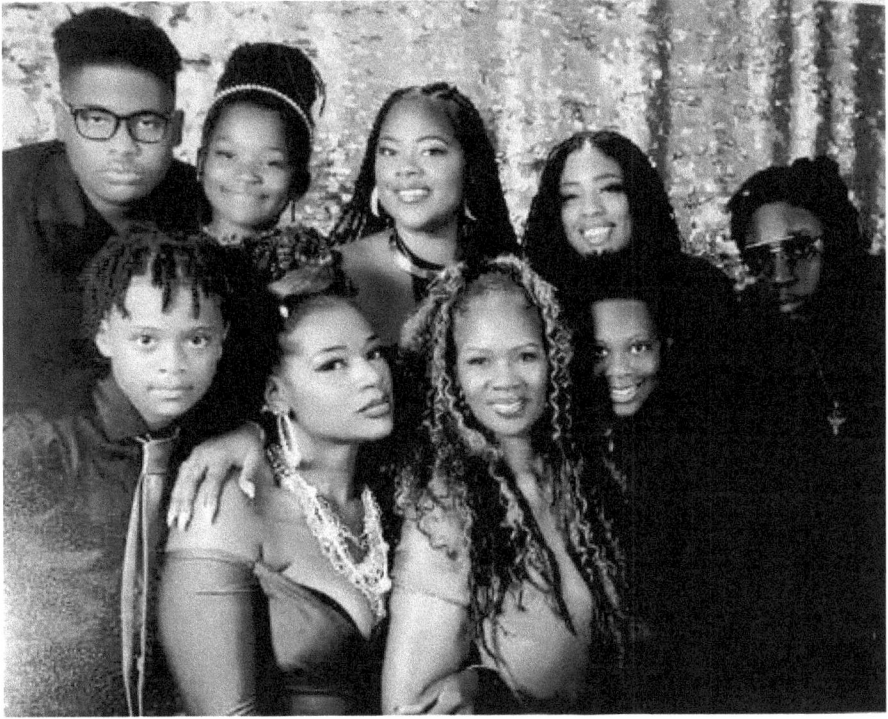

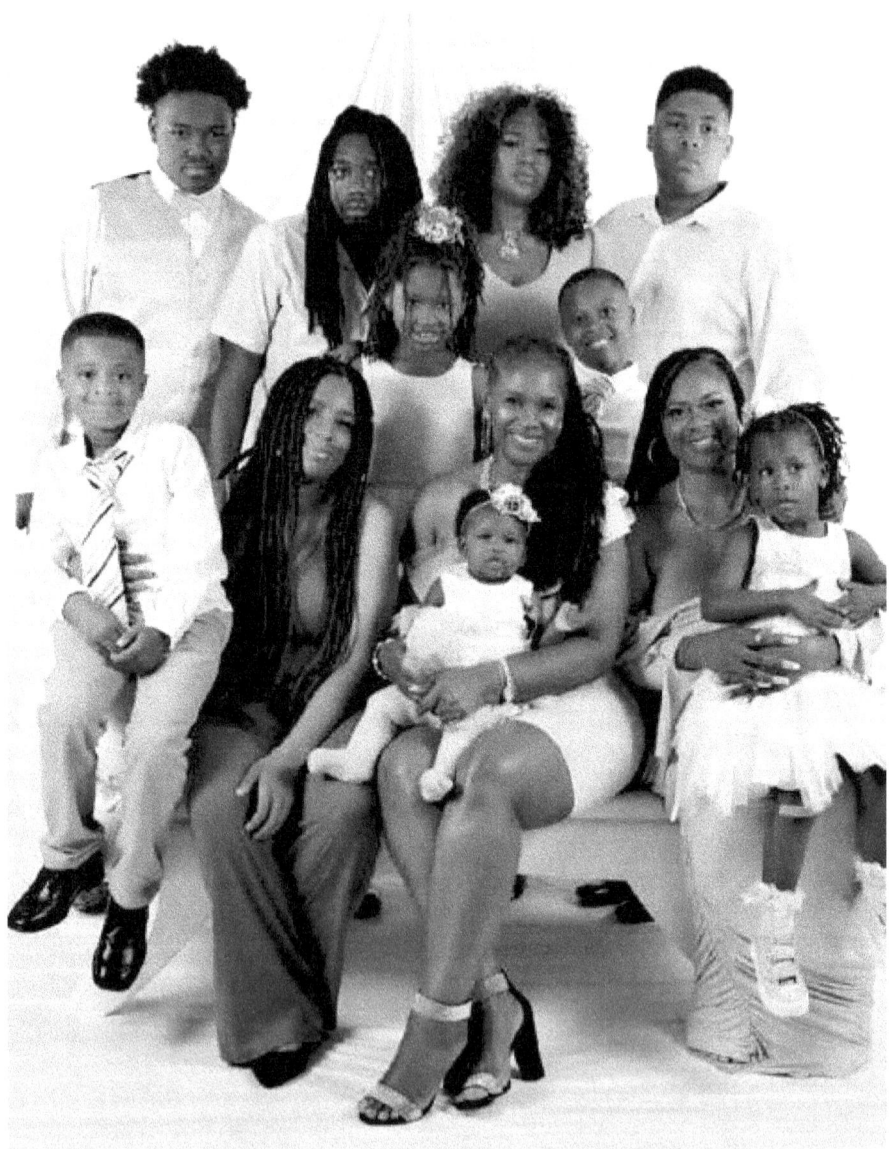

🙏 About The Author 🙏

Dr. Kellie Diane is a Registered Nurse, Ordained Minister, Spiritual Counselor, Entrepreneur, and Servant Leader. She is the CEO of Dr. Kellie Diane LLC and AwareHerness : The Power to Know Personal Development Services. Dr. Kellie is a proud mother of five children and seven grandchildren as well as an aunt and sister.

Dr. Kellie has a special passion for awakening, enlightening, and empowering women to walk in their divine purpose by healing their past wounds. She is particularly drawn to inspiring women and children who have been physically, mentally, and/or sexually abused.

In *Dr. Kellie's* early elementary school years, a teacher recognized her quick learning ability and decided to place her into a higher grade level, in which she successfully excelled without any difficulties. It was then that her English teacher recognized her unique talent for writing and asked her to write and present her very first poetry piece.

It was then that she received her first award for her work at the incredibly young age of nine. Her passion for writing and for inspiring and motivating individuals led her to pursue her dreams of becoming an author, motivational speaker, and mentor.

She has used her platform on several news channels, radio shows, and social media outlets to speak out specifically against social injustices, inequalities, and various women's empowerment topics.

She has been a co-author in various books and magazine articles, spreading messages of healing, awareness, and self-love.

Dr. Kellie has an intense passion for helping individuals navigate through tough times and has used her platform to help others experiencing similar life-changing journeys.

In 1995, she gave birth to a son who was subsequently diagnosed with Autism around the age of 13, prompting her to start "Divinely Connected," a non-profit organization assisting individuals with resources to navigate special needs children. Prior to her son's birth, *Dr. Kellie* spent years caring for special needs adults full-time while in nursing school. She used the skills that she learned to successfully navigate her son through multiple medical specialists, school systems, and behavioral therapists. Her son graduated from high school at the top of his class in Computer Sciences.

In 1997, Dr. Diane completed her Senior Practicum in University of Maryland Medical Center Neonatal Intensive Care Unit where she learned to care for critically ill premature infants, many of which were under one pound. In 2006, *Dr. Kellie* gave birth to her own 1 pound baby girl. Because of her intense training in the Neonatal Unit, she then started a business assisting individuals of premature babies with resources, named Little Miracles Resources and Solutions. Dr. Kellie was able to successfully care for her daughter through various surgeries and hospital admissions. Her daughter is now 17 years old and in college.

Dr. Kellie was the Chief Financial Officer of the First Maryland chapter of "BLACK NURSES ROCK," where she volunteered her skills to oversee all the Maryland chapter's financial needs and obligations. She played a pivotal role in the launching, marketing, and of the development of the now second largest Black nurses organization.

Dr. Kellie has spent hundreds of hours volunteering in the community for Big Brothers/Big Sisters, Camp Holiday Trails, health fairs, mentoring programs, Toys for Tots, and other various programs. She believes that giving back to the community is a great way to motivate, inspire, and encourage individuals to maintain social interaction and psychological well-being.

She is a member of Chi Eta Phi Incorporated, Alpha Kappa Mu National Honor Society and Golden Key International Honor Society.

In her spare time, she loves to cruise, read, write, and spend time with her children and grandchildren. She loves animals and sitting with nature while meditating. Her future goals include writing a sequel to Soul Wounds, international touring, and assisting individuals in starting businesses and leaving legacies.

Dr. Kellie's message to the world is that the process of determination, preservation, and overcoming is still in effect and makes up the fabric of the warrior woman that she is today and will continue to evolve into. Her goal is to continue to awaken women by reminding them that even though the road may seem hopeless, to never give up. That if their journey remains in a perpetual forward motion they are not lost but BECOMING.

Dr. Kellie Diane was born in Richmond, VA, and was subsequently raised in Baltimore, MD.

She holds a Bachelor of Science in Nursing, Master's in Business Administration with an emphasis in Healthcare Administration, a Doctorate in Divinity, and a PHD in Pastoral Counseling.